The Yeoman Diet

by Larsen Halleck

If you're reading this book, you're likely interested in losing weight. If you are, you're not alone---as this country continues to be the dying, decadent empire that it is, it's people are continuing to get more and more embarrassingly fat. You've probably tried various plans and schemes to lose weight, ranging from the simple to the needlessly complicated, and no matter what sort of schemata, cleanse, purge, or lifestyle change you've tried, it just didn't work.

You're probably at the end of your rope and utterly dejected---weight loss just seems like such a complicated thing, right?

Wrong.

Dieting and weight loss are incredibly easy if you look at the problem from a different paradigm. The key, I have found is not to look at the issue from a standpoint of counting calories and nutrient micromanaging, but rather from an issue of *survival*; namely, to *put yourself in a situation of eating to survive and go about your day, and spending an equivalent amount of money on food.*

Does that sound needlessly obtuse? I would assume so, but the next 65 pages will hopefully elaborate on what I mean. And don't just assume that this is idle conjecture---my time as a starving student at CSU San Francisco led me to develop this dietary plan almost by accident: a diet and exercise scheme that made me drop 40 pounds without even knowing it, and gave me a lean and chiseled physique the co-eds could barely keep their hands off of.

It was just that easy for me, and once you've read this book, you'll understand how easy it can be for you as well. All you have to do is take inspiration from your hardscrabble, dirt-farming ancestors, as ridiculous as that may sound. Be like me, and eat like a peasant!

-Larsen

Chapter 1: "...No, really, are you serious?"

If you've read this far, you've probably reacted to the phrase "Eat like a peasant" with shock, horror, pompous laughter, dull incomprehension, or any combination of those things. After all, why would *anybody* want to eat like a peasant? I mean, *everybody* knows that everybody except for royalty was a peasant until, like, yesterday, and those peasants were pustule-faced imbeciles that spent 26 out of every 24 hours laboring for some feudal landlord while they were afflicted with scurvy, rickets, gingivitis, herpes, gonorrhea, hypocalcemia, and about 500 different plagues. Right?

First of all, the term "Eat like a peasant" is more of an analogy or metaphor to give you a rough idea of how the diet works, rather than literally telling you to eat a diet of small beer, blood pudding, and jellied eels.

But more importantly, the diet and lifestyle of the medieval peasant, while not what we in modern times would call "comfortable", was not quite as bad as you've been taught in school, and, speaking strictly in terms of lifestyle and diet (ie: not taking into account the obvious technological and medical advantages), might have some *advantages* over our modern lives, or at the very least have some helpful advice we can glean.

For starters, the medieval peasant paid a much lower tax burden than the modern wageslave[i], had much more vacation time[ii], *ius primae noctis* *probably* didn't actually exist, and his food can probably be said to be equal to the food the modern wageslave consumes: sure, the modern man probably has much more protein, but his food is also full of high fructose corn syrup and soy and lacking in the vital micronutrients that are often lost in the refining of foodstuffs, which, combined with a lack of exercise, can in some extreme cases makes him simultaneously obese and malnourished. Indeed, archaeological evidence would suggest that in some respects their dentition was *healthier* than the modern man---they certainly would have been missing teeth, but the lack of refined sugars meant that the teeth they had were strong and healthy.

If that weren't enough, some researchers, notably Gold University's Peter McAllister, have remarked that osteological evidence suggests that the ancients would have been much, *much* stronger and more physically capable than the modern man---namely, the thickness of the diaphyses (shafts) of ancient long bones are much thicker than their modern counterparts, and the muscle attachments are comparably larger as well (ie: two parts of a bone that are affected by ontogenetic forces much more than congenital forces). Or, to put it in layman's terms, only the most elite of Olympic archers can pull the 15th century English longbow, a weapon that was by definition a weapon of the "yeoman", which is to say a free landowner holding less than 100 acres of land. In other words, a peasant[iii].

Are you starting to feel a little inferior?

So having read that little diatribe, the smarter of my readers are likely starting to figure out what the basic premise of the "peasant weight loss plan" is. If that is the case, feel free to put the book down and implement it. Bear in mind that I don't consider myself to be "the smarter of" most groups of people, so I understand if you need to have things explicitly explained to you.

The basic premise of this weight loss plan is to combine the physical activity levels of the medieval/early Renaissance Yeoman (which is to say nigh-constant and ranging in intensity level from moderate to insanely strenuous) with a diet that gives you all of the vital nutrients you need in sensible portions by eating "common sense" foodstuffs---in short a diet that combines the variety and convenience of modernity with the simplicity and cost-effectiveness of our ancient forebears that had to scrounge for every calorie and count every farthing and gilder.

Are you still confused? Worry not, all of this will be explained in the following chapters. Note the short length of this book---all the concepts of this diet are very easily explained for even the densest of readers in less than 70 pages.

If you don't believe me, just take a look at myself: Like I said in the foreword, I lost 40 pounds on this diet without even worrying about losing weight: weight loss and low stress? What more can you want?

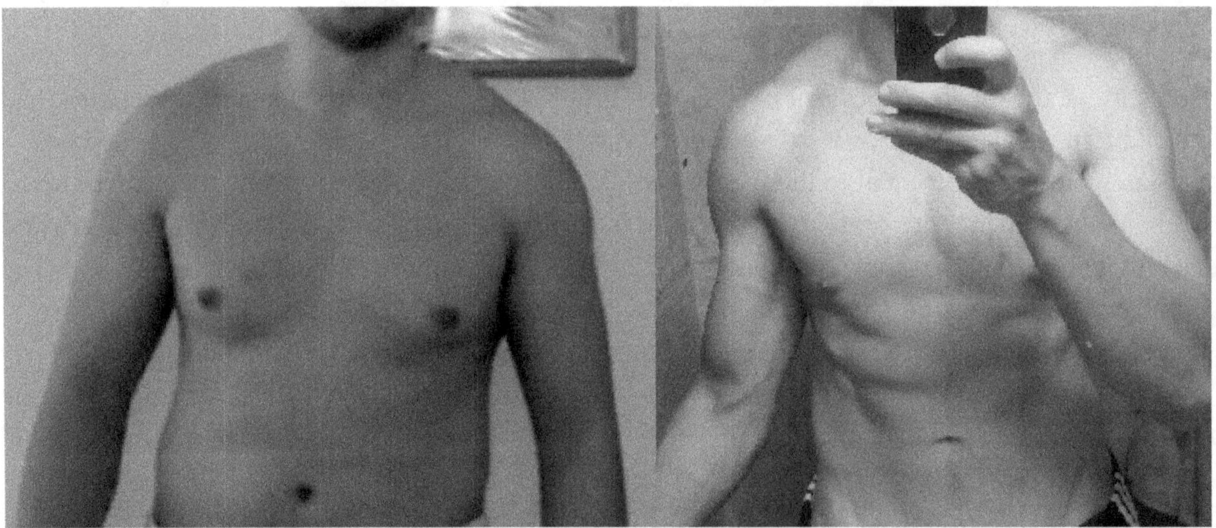

Left: 215 Right: 176

Chapter 2: Diet is the easiest thing

The key in "eating like a peasant" is to sort of mentally put yourself into the mindset of being a hardscrabble dirt farmer who needs to stay alive while conserving as much of your resources as possible. In layman's terms, the first thing you have to do is imbibe the concept of **<u>eating to save money.</u>**

I underlined it and bolded it, that's how important it is. If you understand this concept, combined with what foods are healthy and what foods are not healthy, I guarantee that you will not only lose weight, but you'll lose weight without even realizing you lose weight. By far, this is the most important concept you have to understand for this diet to work,

I'll go out on a limb here and say that, for general purposes of health and well-being, you do not need to spend more than 200 dollars a month on groceries, and every cent of that 200 dollars can be put into good, healthy, nourishing food. Remember, you're a peasant, you have to conserve what little you have while also making your body function.

And <u>please</u>, before we get into how to do this, spare me any whiny fatbody diatribes about how "it's so hard to eat healthy food in America, muh food deserts", and so forth. By the time you finish this chapter, you'll never sling that excuse again.

Here's how it works:

When you go grocery shopping, bring only 100 dollars with you, and not a penny more. Then purchase food for all three meals of the day. Here is my own shopping list, you don't necessarily have to use this, but I think this will illustrate the "don't eat crap" diet better than anything else. If you want other suggestions for what to eat, check the appendix for a few sample meal plans that I have given to my clients in my day job as a personal trainer.

Breakfast Essentials:

Eggs

Bacon

Oatmeal (preferably steel cut, not machine cut)

Two packs of "accessory Fruit" (blueberries, grapes, strawberries, small fruit you can put in the oatmeal. Perhaps figs or dates if you're feeling exotic)

Lunch Essentials:

One loaf of bread (make it last two weeks)

Lunch Meat (one pack, make it last)

One unit of cheese (good proppa cheese, make it last)

Some sort of brined preserve (pickles, artichoke hearts, olives, accessories to the lunch. One jar!)

Hand fruits of many types (apples, oranges, bananas, pears, und so weiter). Between 12 and 24 units (one fruit=one unit).

Dinner essentials:

Green vegetables (your mustard greens, your spinach, green beans, asparagus, and so forth). Fresh or frozen or canned

Meats (personally I would buy 2 pounds of ground beef for two weeks of post workout meals. In addition, units of chicken wings and legs, pork chops, fish, sausage, possibly organ meats if they're available. Usually not steak, shit is expensive. Eyeball it to determine how much you need-and remember you can halve things.)

Complex carbohydrates (brown rice, noodles, semolina, etc. Buy a multiple pound bag, this'll last you at least a month if you're smart about it)

Non-Perishables/Snacks/Others

Cans of fish in oil (buy a few with each shopping trip, they last for years and thus you put them in the cabinet)

Brined preserves (so important you gotta do it again, buy one or two)

Canned soups, vegetables, beans (it's good shit)

Another bag of rice or dried noodles

Mixed nuts and trail mix (non-perishable snack, make it last! Also get the kind that doesn't have chocolate in it, numbnuts)

Salt

Baking Powder

Flour (for hardtack)

At most this will cost 100 dollars, and will last you two weeks with judicious rationing. For added fun, try to get your prices down as low as possible---some days I've even managed to buy two weeks worth of grocery for 75 dollars.

This rough-hewn dietary plan will provide all of the macronutrients (protein, carbs, and fat) you need to function, and most of the micronutrients as well (vitamins and minerals), and it's cheap.

Some, of course, would argue that you can buy a lot more crappy food for the same price, but again the aim is to eat healthily and cheaply.

A good rule of thumb for purchasing food is to ask yourself "Would a man from the year 1900 recognize this as food?" Or to put it another way, "would somebody from the year 1400 recognize this as food?" If not, it's probably not something you should be eating. Rates of obesity, heart disease, and other objective measures of bad health were much lower in the gilded age then they are now, to say nothing of a few centuries before that. Avoid junk food, or overly processed food, keep it simple, and you should be fine. And if you really need help on what food is healthy and what food is not healthy, go to a dietician, they'll likely have free pamphlets that will give you all the information you could ever possibly need.

You've gone to public school, you've seen the food pyramid---it's not bad, which is rare to say for a government program, but in fact the government has made some good efforts in reducing obesity (I suppose the USG realizes that a nation of lardasses will not be productive laborers). Just eat this, and you'll more or less get all the nutrients you need.

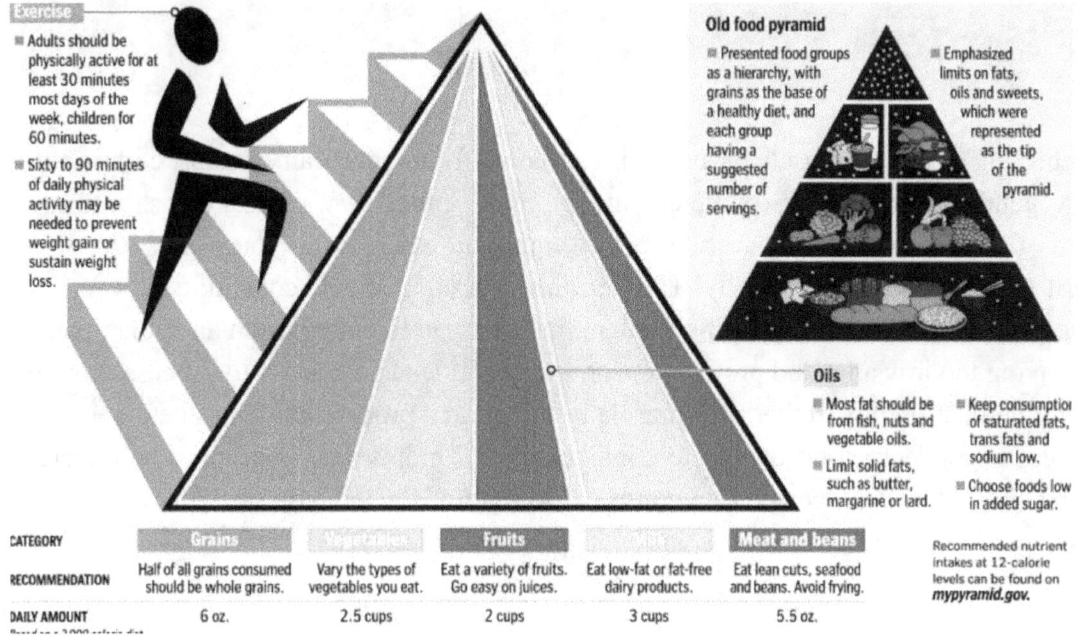

If I had to sum up what a healthful diet is for 99% of the population, all I need is three words: "Don't. Eat. Shit."---use common sense, and like I said above, don't eat what Great-Grandpa wouldn't recognize.

Note that I repeatedly said that the food you've purchased should last you two weeks, and that's another major tenet of the weightloss program---judicious rationing of food to save money and calories!

To put it simply, EAT LESS FOOD. You don't need nearly as much food as you think you do. A good way of rationing food that I have discovered is to eat "from the palm of your hand". What this means is that all your units of food should fit in the palm of your hand. IE: Your vegetables should fit in the palm of your hand, your meat, and your carbs. That's a meal, low in calories and low in price, while still giving you all of the necessary nutrients to function.

Does that sound a little bland? It can be, but you can throw various condiments and spices on it to liven things up a bit. Since you're trying to lose weight, you're going to have to prioritize nutrition and cutting calories over being a gourmand. You can't have everything in life, deal with it.

That will all suffice for purposes of simply losing weight and retaining a good amount of muscle mass. But if you want to pack on _more_ muscle mass, you will have to increase your total caloric consumption (obviously, to gain any sort of weight whether it be muscle or adipose tissue you have to eat more calories and spend more money...or you can shoplift all your food like some people that are _not_ named Larsen Halleck do. Damn those handsome devils!)

Of those calories, you have to eat a certain percentage of each macronutrient (remember, the macros, the most important nutrients for total systemic health are protein, fat, and carbohydrates).

Protein:

The main "building block" of muscle tissue. This can come from meat, dairy, beans, certain types of fruit and vegetables, and of course supplements. To make things _very_ simple, you should eat about 1 gram of protein per each kilogram of bodyweight you weigh (ie: if you weigh 100 kilograms eat 100 grams of protein) daily. Those grams of protein should constitute between 20-35% of your total caloric intake daily---higher than that can lead to dehydration and constipation issues (and having too low a fat and protein consumption will lead your body to process proteins for glucose for cellular energy, rather than muscle building, in a process known as ketosis). In general, as long as you keep your total protein intake below 2 grams per kilogram of bodyweight, you should be okay. Between one and two grams per kilogram is where you want to be to put on muscle mass.

Carbohydrates:

Simple sugars, starches/complex sugars, and fiber (non-digestible carbohydrates that still provide a non-nutrient benefit).

In general, you want to eat complex carbohydrates (brown rice, fruits and vegetables) more than simple sugars (table sugar and the like)---they have more nutrients than just carbohydrates and they have fiber which improves colonic health and increases feelings of satiation, while still ultimately providing you with the glucose fix that keeps every part of your body functioning. And with that cellular energy, you will have the capacity to exercise longer. "Fat burns in a carbohydrate flame", after all.

You should consume roughly 6-8 grams of carbohydrates per kilogram of bodyweight, and total carbohydrate consumption should be 45-60% of your total caloric consumption (this combined with the increased protein consumption detailed above). Before you panic in reading that statistic, remember that the key is *percentage*. The only "Secret" to losing weight is to decrease the total caloric consumption across the board.

Fat:

A group of compounds that include triglycerides (fatty acids, fats and oils), phospholipids, and sterols. Of dietary lipids, 95% are triglycerides, and in the body 99% of stored lipids are triglycerides. Structurally, triglycerides are three fatty acids attached to a glycerol backbone.

Polyunsaturated fatty acids are essential fatty acids (or fats that cannot be manufactured by the body but are essential for proper health/function). Those saturated fatty acids you always hear about are implicated as a risk factor for heart disease because they raise the bad cholesterol (LDL, low density lipoprotein) levels. Unsaturated fats are associated with good cholesterol (high density lipoprotein, HDL) increases and decreased risk of heart disease. Trans fats are effectively similar to the saturated fats. However, do bear in mind that for men especially, saturated fats are a dietary necessity despite their risks due to the body using them to produce sterols and androgens---so for saturated fats eat the recommended daily allowance and not any more.

Fats are used in long term energy storage and as carriers for many vitamins. They also form cellular membranes (among other things), so they are *vital* for bodily functions.

The Acceptable Macronutrient Distribution Range (AMDR) for fat intake is 20-35% of the total calorie intake---but seeing as there doesn't seem to be too many negative effects of having fat consumption between 10-20%, err on the side of eating less fat than more. Since fats are calorically dense (ie: small amounts have high calories), you can overeat fats very easily, so watch out! In general, if you're eating sufficient amounts of protein and carbohydrates like I detailed above, you'll likely be getting enough fats, so you don't need to worry about this.

If you're eating actual food (ie: not supplements) to get those nutrients in sufficient quantities, then by definition you're going to be getting all the necessary micronutrients as well (your vitamins and inorganic nutrients and etc.)---eating wholesome meats and dairy will give you B and D vitamins and inorganic nutrients like iron and calcium, fruits and vegetables will give you the water soluble vitamins, foods with healthy fats will give you the fat soluble vitamins, etc.

And that's really all that needs to be said about diet---I will repeat myself: it is BY FAR the simplest part of this program. Things are more complicated ahead, so, as your skirt wearing ancestors likely would have said, "Gird your loins".

Chapter 3: Exercise and Science, together at last!

Now we get into exercise, which is going to provide the lion's share of your weight loss. But before we can go into exercise programming, we have to discuss the science behind it, so you can have some idea of what your arduous labors will be affecting, and which exercises are effective and which are not.

Before we begin, I want you to learn a very important concept: a good exercise routine should not involve any more than 10 different resistance exercises, and should not take more than an hour and a half a day *at most*. If anybody tells you otherwise (more often than not, it will be something about the amount of exercises you're doing), they're trying to sell you something. And don't worry about what a "Resistance exercise" is, we'll get to that in a second.

Another fundamental concept you must realize to train effectively is that: all the worthwhile "hardware" innovations for physical training were invented by 1905: 1905 being the year that Thomas Inch of the United Kingdom invented the plate loading barbell.

(To be more specific, that should read "all of the hardware innovations FOR OTHERWISE HEALTHY PEOPLE. Since becoming a certified personal trainer, I have gotten more experience working with those who are somewhat invalid, and thus I give them leeway with regards to using machines since they are not physically capable of doing any free weights. If possible, you should always err on the side of free weights, since they are superior for developing functional strength, coordination, and balance).

Even the most casual observer, whose only experience with physical training is watching 80s action movies can tell you there's more than one type of way to be physically adroit. More accurately, there are three, speaking purely in terms of muscular and/or nervous system function (so this does not include hand-to-eye coordination or other skills related to team sports). These variants are dependent upon certain types of muscle fibers, and their correlation to axon action of the Central and Peripheral nervous system. You can see this whenever you eat chicken-you have the white meat, and the dark meat. Those are different types of muscle that correlate to different parts of the chicken's body.

The dark meat is found in the legs-red muscle, or slow oxidative, is a type of muscle fiber that slowly contracts (as commanded by the axons, which are, to put it very simply, extensions of neurons, the basic cells of the nervous system, that connect to various parts of the body, and send electrical impulses based on other electrical impulses from both the brain and the external environment) and slowly produces lactic acid (the stuff that causes "the burn", to tell you when you're over-exerting yourself).

It is found in the legs for obvious reasons, the chicken spends most of its day walking around, thus needing that stamina. This is the type of muscle fiber that is found in endurance athletes-such as marathoners. Note that muscular endurance (ie: your legs not getting tired in a marathon) corroborates directly with cardiovascular endurance.

The white meat is what is dubbed "fast glycolytic" muscle. This is, as one might expect by contrasting the previous paragraph, a muscle fiber that quickly and powerfully contracts in a bout of maximal exertion. In accordance with its power, these muscles quickly and abundantly produce lactic acid, a hormone that acts in a positive feedback reaction-i.e.: your body telling you to take it easy or you'll tear something. This type of meat is found in the breast and wings, because the chicken cannot sustain flight, and has no need to-just a quick sprint to get away from predators. This type of muscle is found in any athlete that needs a quick burst of power-sprinters, Olympic weightlifters, ring gymnasts, etc.

 (Bear in mind I have highly simplified this, and there are other types of muscle fibers, but for our purposes, this information will suffice).

 Training in one way or another will cause your body to generate skeletal muscle tissue that is either white or red, and you cannot have a maximal degree of both (you ever see a marathoner step into the weight room and snatch 400 pounds over his head? Me neither.) Despite that, you would not say that any person with a high degree of either is "unfit".

In addition to the two types of muscular exertion, there's also balance/flexibility/dexterity/grace or whatever you'd like to call it. This is more of the nervous system's bag, corroborating with the inner ear (and its twiddly little sensory hairs that direct a person's sense of balance), a person's innate center of gravity, and one or more of the types of muscle fibers (depending on what it is you're doing) to do a variety of things. An Olympic gymnast differs greatly from a champion ballroom dancer in physical terms, but they would both be described as graceful, flexible and balanced, and are both certainly physically adroit.

And, finally, I've gotten to the point: there we have the three types of physicality-power (encompassing strength and speed), endurance (of both the skeletal muscles and the cardiovascular system), and dexterity (encompassing balance, flexibility, and grace). Think of these not as rigid "compartments", but as something of a Venn diagram. It is impossible to be a world class athlete in all three, but it is quite possible to be above average in all three-an Olympic class men's gymnast is quite capable of deadlifting twice his bodyweight, to cite one example.

Now that all of that science is out of the way, let's get to what you really want to know: the actual exercises themselves. I personally prefer to be something of a "jack of all trades", physically, but the information can be adapted to fit your specific purposes (if you'd want to specialize in one).

In accordance with the above, I split my routine into three facets: the maximum strength routine, the muscular endurance routine, and the cardio/flexibility routine (this confusing dichotomy will be explained below). In addition to these, I have added on what I have dubbed "informal exercise", and combining the previous three (Which we can call "formal exercise") with the "informal exercise" is my secret to weight loss.

But before we can discuss informal exercise, we must discuss "formal" exercise.

<u>What Is Formal Exercise?</u>

(Bear in mind that, despite the fact that I am a personal trainer, I'm pretty sure I am in fact the only person to ever actually use the terms "formal and informal" exercise, mainly because I have never seen "official" terms for these. My reasons will make sense to you once the chapter has been read).

Lover to some, harsh mistress to others, I use the term "formal exercise" to mean exactly what even the most uncoordinated tub thinks of when they hear the term "exercise"---a structured and regimented period of your day when you set aside a period of time solely for physical activity for its own sake, presumably changing into workout-specific clothing. To speak briefly about what sort of clothes you want to be dressing in, you want to be dressing in comfortable, pliant clothing that absorbs sweat and facilitates movement----no burlap, no *vatermorder* stiff collars (for those of you who want to LARP as an actual peasant). T-Shirts, sweatpants, drawstring shorts, sweat socks, and sneakers.

As a rule of thumb I have always argued that to facilitate easy movement the trainee should wear as little clothing as possible---and yes, I <u>would</u> work out in the nude if it were socially acceptable to do so. As an addendum to this: no, fat people, nobody cares what you look like in the gym. Sto using that as an excuse.

Ahem

Anyway, as we discussed previously, there are 3 sorts of athletic "functions" you can train for---and I certainly do. I do not train all three on all days (this is to give the muscles time to recuperate and grow stronger), but nonetheless I do some form of formal exercise 6 days a week, with one day being a day of rest.

My workout schedule as of now is as follows:

Monday: Rest

Tuesday: Weights

Wednesday/Thursday: Cardio

Friday: Calisthenics

Saturday/Sunday: Martial Arts

This provides me with a solid amount of training to make myself a "jack of all trades"---not an elite in one facet or another, but certainly fit enough to do anything I'd desire doing.

Let us go through the list and discuss what each of these mysterious categories is---bear in mind you do not have to use this exact schedule, but for optimal results you must occupy all seven days more or less like this, with extra care to separate resistance training days by at least 48 hours.

<u>WEIGHTS:</u>

Exactly what it sounds like: Exercises in which you carry weights in a way that places great stress upon a certain skeleto-muscular group. You then move said skeleto-muscular group through its complete range of motion in order to induce microfractures/microtears in the bones and muscles, which will then heal in a way that makes the muscle and bone stronger.

In general, free weights should always be done rather than machines, because free weights place greater stress upon the body and due to their inherent instability (*you* put 300 pounds on your back and try to keep your balance!), they work smaller, support muscles (dubbed stabilizers or synergists depending on the movement) often neglected by the machines, which all culminates in greater, more functional strength and agility. Indeed, I often say to my trainees that you shouldn't do any sort of exercise invented after 1905! That being the year Thomas Inch invented the plate loading barbell.

UNLESS you have some sort of balance issue, or arthritis, or some other debilitating health issue. THEN, and only then, will I allow you to use machines. Machines are much easier and simpler to use, and require much less instruction---just work through as deep a range of motion as you can, and keep your form impeccable, and you'll be fine.

If you're not actually handicapped, you have no excuse; nut up and grab the free weights!

As luck would have it, every exercise I advocate here is a *compound* exercise, one that works multiple muscle groups. Thus, you won't need to do more than 10 or so weight exercises---because who wants to spend hour upon hour in the gym?

Also bear in mind I would prefer you to master the calisthenic series on later pages before you start doing weights, but you don't have to heed this advice.

In contrast to the calisthenic exercises, you will never do these for high repetitions: at most, you will be doing 5-6 repetitions in sets of 2 or 3, with a cool down rep afterwards with a lower weight. When you can do this, you increase the weight.

It SHOULD go without saying, but...don't over-exert yourself with weights. It's better to do a low weight with proper form than a gimpy, half-assed heavy weight.

Many weight exercises that I do are just weighted calisthenics: as such, you can learn about those in the corresponding section; just hold a dumbbell in your other hand/between your legs when you do it.

The weight-specific exercises I will teach you are what are colloquially dubbed "the big four" lifts. Combine these with the 6 calisthenic techniques you'll learn later, and you will literally work out every muscle in your body.

1) The Overhead Press

Like all exercises worth doing, there are many variations on this, but for the novice I always recommend the most basic and instinctual movement: The overhead push press.

The push press is one of the best things you can do for development of shoulder strength and size, and the push press is one of the most practical exercises you can do for training for the rigors of daily life-you will rarely lay on your back and push up outside of the gym, but you'll very commonly find the need to lift something over your head, whether it be a box or a friend trying to climb a fence.

 The push press is also known as the "jerk," as in the second component of the Olympic lift known as the "clean and jerk" (the Olympic lifts are a discipline that are even more about technique than they are sheer muscular strength, and as such I do not recommend them for the beginner).

To start, go to a rack or power cage. Place the bar on the rack at chest level and load it up with whatever amount of weight you can handle.

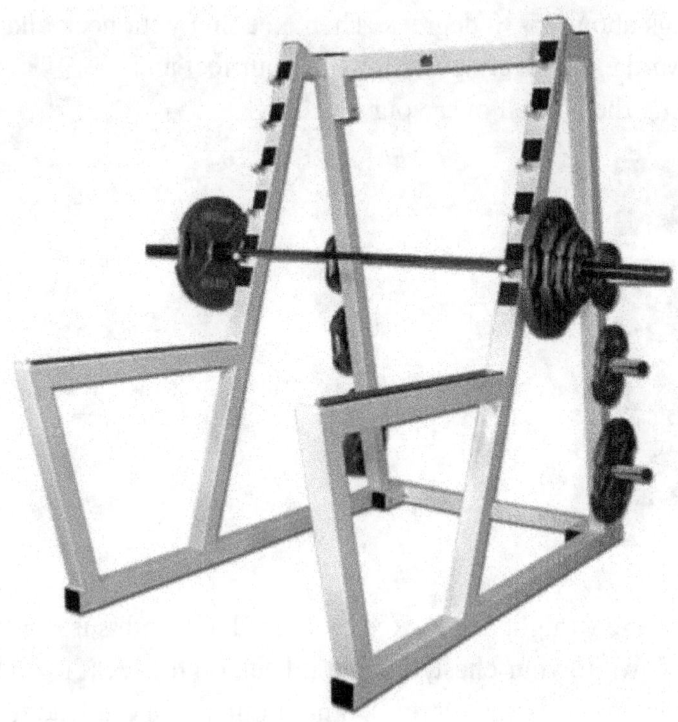

As usual, I will advocate that you start light and do the exercise with proper form.

Take the barbell and hold it to your chest. This is the start position.

Some lifters prefer to keep their wrists locked and forward as seen on the left of the picture below, and some prefer to roll their wrists back slightly and roll them forward on the lift. I will advise you to just do whichever feels natural to you (I find that rolling the wrists back forces the collarbone to bear some of the weight, and thus makes me lift slightly more, but if you choose this, don't roll them back too much!

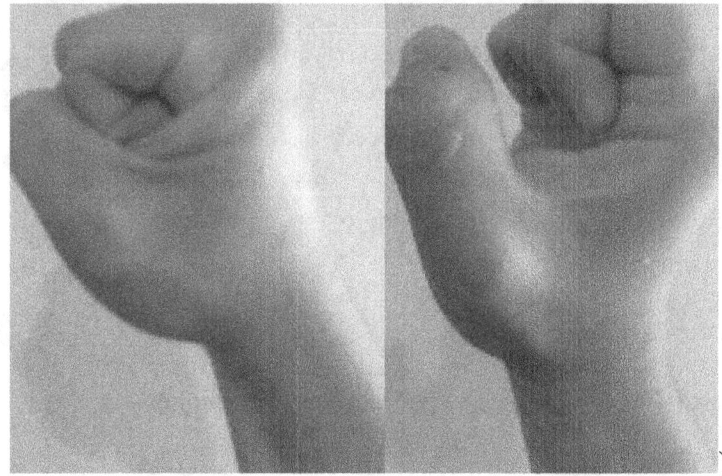
)

Beginning in the start position, bend the legs about 25-30 degrees. Then, keeping your neck and back tight and straight, and your head forward explosively push up with your feet and simultaneously push up with the arms, lifting the barbell over your head.

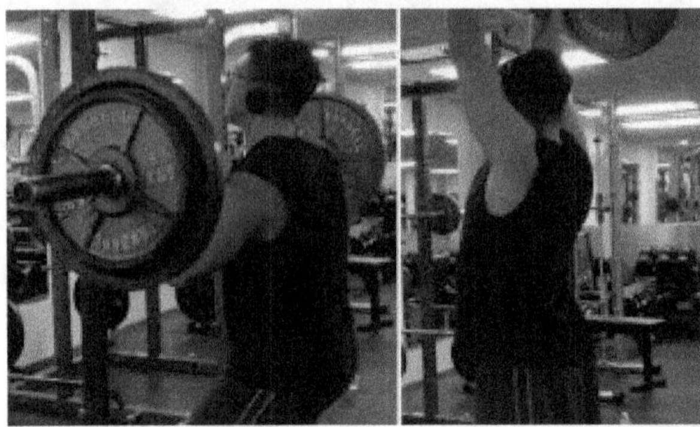

Yours truly with 215 pounds

The lift is not properly done unless the arms are straight and locked over head. Once this is done, slowly and under control bring the weight down to your chest, and put it back on the rack. I cannot emphasize enough that you must "dismount" with control. Doing it otherwise can lead to serious injury.

2) The Bench Press

Some fitness trainers disparage the bench press, seeing it as less practical than other presses. And they're right. The association with archetypal "dudebros" hasn't helped the bench press's reputation either. However, while it is not the MOST practical, it's still worth doing, and is advocated by strength athletes such as Olympic shotputters. Or in the words of Pavel Tsatsouline "For all the debate over the usefulness of the bench press, if you met someone with a 600 pound bench press, would you want to take a punch from them?"

The bench press will develop the pectorals, triceps, and shoulders predominantly, with some auxiliary work done for the forearms and hands. I will be teaching you the standard, shoulder width bench press with a "closed grip." It will serve most of your pectoral training needs, particularly when done in conjunction with other upper body exercises (as a side note, I only do the standard bench press, since unlike your average "upper body day every day" gym stereotype, I have a day job and thus time is of the essence).

As with the overhead press, there are a couple of rules for proper form.

1) The bar must GENTLY touch the chest before going back up. Gentleness is the key for reasons that are so obvious, I don't think they have to be gone over.

2) throughout any type of bench press, the feet should be pressing down hard on the floor, causing the back to slightly arch-and I emphasize SLIGHTLY. This will give you a little bit of a

"boost" in your lifting and enable you to lift a few pounds more than you could have otherwise thanks to the magic of proprioceptive muscular tension, which I have published articles about on the internetix

3) Get a spotter. I normally don't work out with a partner, but the bench press needs a partner for the obvious reason that failing a bench press leaves an un-liftable weight planted firmly on your chest.

So now that that's cleared up: to do the bench press, you start by finding a bench.

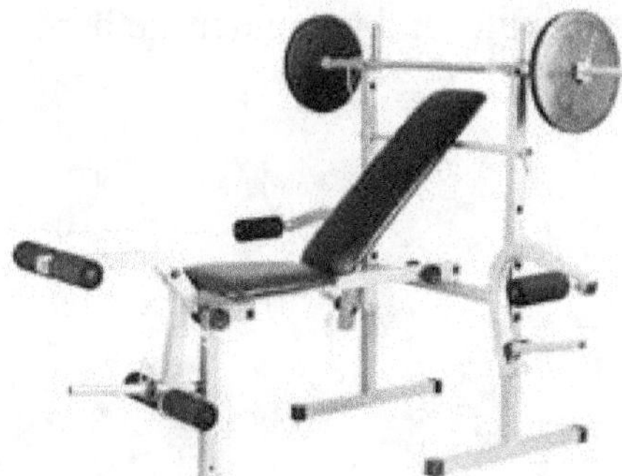

Once you have found the bench, place the bar on the top rung of platforms, and place yourself under the bar, approximately so the bar is directly over the top of your pectoral muscles. Placing the bar on its highest setting will make starting the exercise easier, rather than expending effort on something that is not actually part of the exercise.

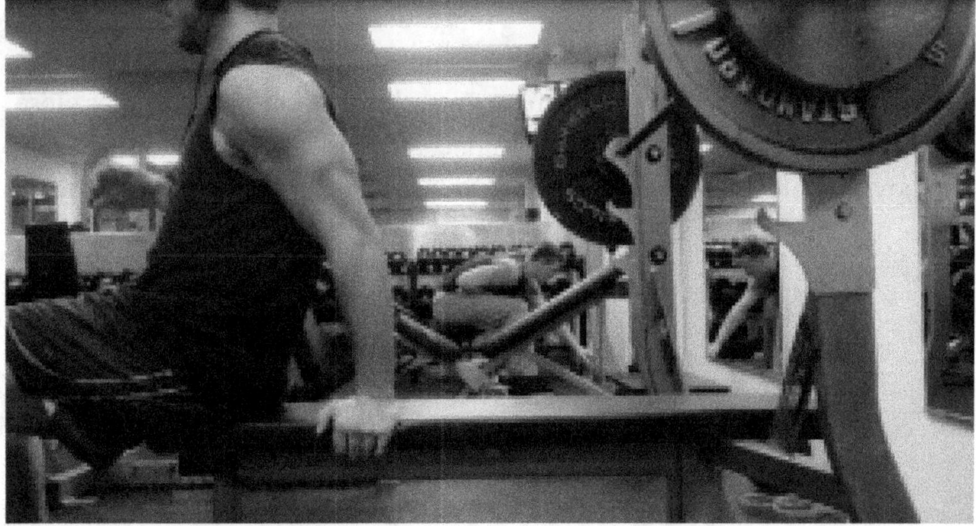

The bar can be held with a variety of grips, but for beginners I would advocate just a regular fist grip, also called the "closed grip." Just hold the bar naturally, with the four fingers around the bar and the thumb clenching the fingers. Let the hands find the position they want to find, push down hard with your feet to arch your back, and then push up with your arms and hold the bar over your head. This is the start position.

Once you've lifted the bar into the start position, keeping the feet pressing throughout the entirety of the exercise, lower the bar down in a smooth, controlled motion, touch the chest

GENTLY, and bring it back up to the start position. As with the overhead press, this is a maximal strength exercise, so an enormous amount of reps is not required.

Also bear in mind that if you are interested purely in aesthetics (And if you're seeking to lose weight, then you *are)*, the incline bench press should also be done to give size and definition to the upper pectorals, giving you the nice rounded pectorals you always see in the magazines.

To do the incline bench, imply adjust the bench to a 20-45 degree angle, and get under the bar as shown

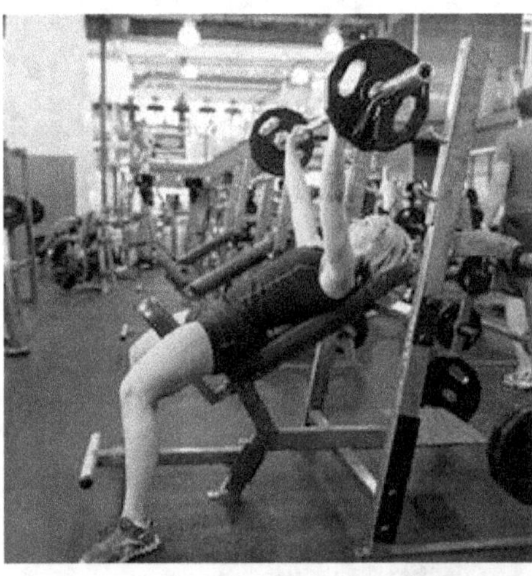

Then perform a bench press---obviously you cannot do the same amount of weight with this then with a standard bench press, so lower the weight. Keeping your elbows tight and tucked as close to the body as you can, bring the bar down to your collar bone, and push up. If you do this exercise wrong, your elbows will feel it *immediately*. So if you don't feel pain, you know you're doing it right.

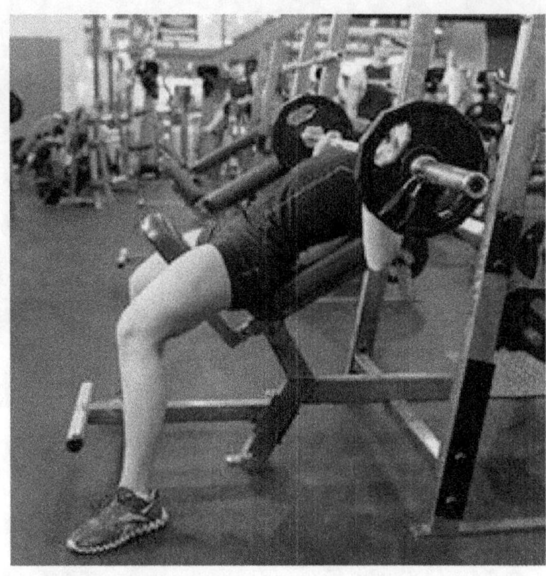

3) The Deadlift

I have repeatedly gone on record saying that when it comes to weightlifting, there are only four lift exercises that you absolutely need to do, and this opinion is shared by many other fitness coaches and fitness enthusiasts.

Now, having gone over the upper body half of the "big four", we must of course learn how to exercise the lower body. To be a truly strong and fit man, you have to work out your lower body as well, in a way that will make your legs, waist, hips, and core both functional and aesthetically pleasing. And, as luck would have it there are only two simple-but-difficult exercises you need: the squat and the deadlift.

And while they're both very useful, I would recommend the deadlift as the more important of the two, because while the squat will hit every muscle below and including the lower back, the deadlift will hit 90% of those same muscles, and provide a pretty solid exercise for the upper body as well. More specifically, the deadlift will predominantly hit the trapezius muscles and the muscles of the forearm and hands. And you can read my online articles if you want to see how much importance I place on forearm training.

The first thing you absolutely need to learn in order to to do the deadlift is how to "hollow" the back, or as I prefer to call it, "lock" the back. This technique keeps the back tight and straight during the deadlift, which is imperative to do because otherwise you risk severe back injury.

Stand with your feet shoulder width apart, then exaggeratedly "Stand at attention"---imagine your body lengthening and straightening like a soldier in an old cartoon (laugh if you must, this metaphor helped me visualize the proper position). Feel your chest puff out and your lower back tense. This back tightness is the feeling you want to maintain throughout the deadlift.

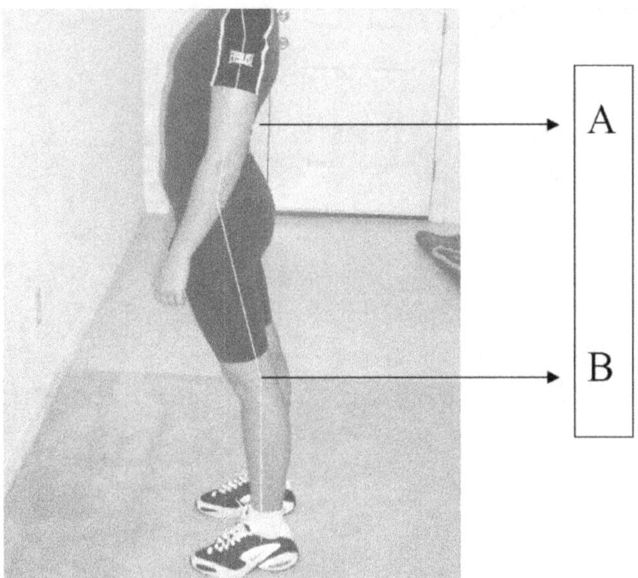

This is from a medical text showing the pathology known as hyperlordosis, but for purposes of "locking" the back, I feel it helps as a visual aid.

Once you have familiarized yourself with that feeling, you can do the deadlift. Place the bar on the floor and load it with whatever weights you need. Roll the bar to your shins. Then lock the back, keep the head and neck tight and looking forward---this helps with proper spinal alignment. While maintaining this locked position, keep your arm straight and begin bending at the knees to the bar. Do what feels natural and bend until your hands can grip the bar. Do not bend at the back or move your shoulders or anything.

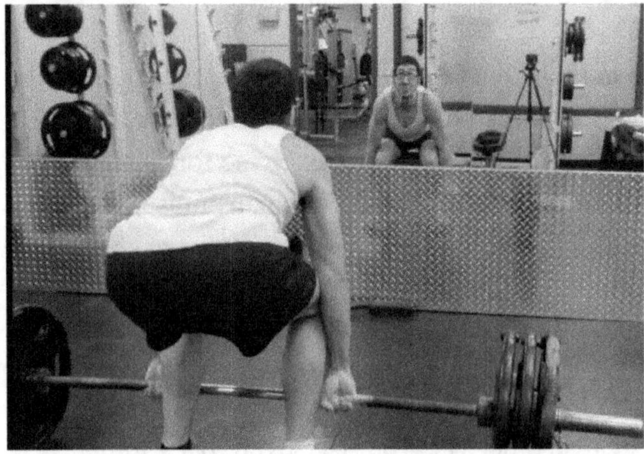

The picture is of yours truly, biting the bullet and using the slightly mortifying ass shot to demonstrate proper form

Then begin lifting, maintain the total body tightness and begin lifting with your legs. You should feel as if you are pushing through the floor, which is why I recommend that you do this barefoot--assuming you don't need a medical orthotic like your illustrious trainer (me) still does.

Push from the floor and the weight should begin to move. Continue pushing until your legs are straight as shown in the picture. The bar should be about at your knees.

Then, clench the buttocks and straighten out at the back and hips, making sure to keep them both tight. The bar should finish at about your hip level.

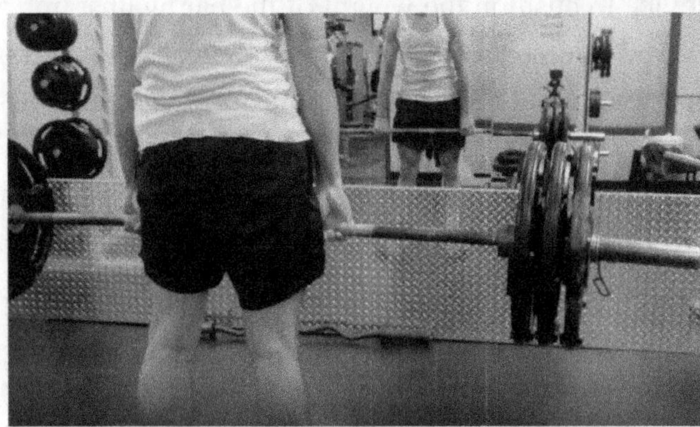

To release the weight, do NOT drop the weights like an asshole. Instead, just do a reversal of the lifting motion. Lock the back and bend at the waist until the bar reaches your knees. Then bend at the knees until the bar touches the ground.

I have said this before, but it bears repeating: form is imperative! I give this advice especially for the deadlift, as improper form can lead to slipped discs and broken backs. The bridging you will learn later can only protect you so much. If you feel any pain in doing this exercise, whether it be in your back or your hips, stop immediately, lower the weight, and work on your form.

4) The Squat

The squat is arguably the best exercise for the legs, and inarguably a fundamental motion for any athlete or physical culturist. This is because doing the squat properly will not only train the big muscles of the quadriceps, but also the calves, the feet, the buttocks, and the hips. Combine this with the deadlift (which hits the hamstrings much better than the squat), and you'll never need any other lower body exercises. And it goes without saying that in training your legs, you'll make yourself run faster, jump higher, punch and kick harder, grapple stronger, and do anything you want to do better. From the lumbo-pelvic-hip complex comes ALL movement.

To do this exercise, you will need a rack or power cage, preferably the latter as it has safety bars to put the weight down should you be incapable of lifting the weight. To begin, remove the archetypal dudebro doing curls in the squat rack---you're a man and you've got real exercises to do!

Once that's been done, place the bar in the rack at about shoulder/neck level. Load it with whatever amount of weight you wish.

Then, duck under the bar and then stand up straight, with the bar rest on your trapezius muscles and shoulders---NOT your neck---and gripping the bar with an overhand grip, which you should recall from the pull-up section.

Some lifters with a little bit of experience might be asking why I don't advocate using the pad, or that weird ox-yolk thing, or any other sort of device to cushion the weight of the bar against my shoulders. The reason is that I'm not a little girl, and I don't need to protect my delicate shoulders with a "pussy pad". Grab the bar, flex your upper back, and suck it up. If your form is right, you don't need the pad.

Having grasped the bar properly, you must get yourself ready to lift. Get yourself comfortable and place your feet shoulder width apart. Look straight ahead and lock/hollow the back. If that sounds familiar, it should---it's the exact same preparatory steps you took to do the deadlift. This speaks to the shared muscles these exercises target, and the shared risk for injury should form be improperly done.

However, while back injury is a possibility with the squat, the knees and ankles are much more at risk, and will be discussed shortly.

Anyway, keep your feet pointing straight ahead or slightly pointed out. This keeps the knees from pronating inward, which is not something you want to be doing---it weakens the squat and leads to risk of injury.

Begin squatting down in a controlled fashion, while keeping your torso tight and your feet angled properly. Squat down at least until your hips are parallel to your knees, and preferably until your hamstrings touch your calves---or "ass to grass" as the laymen say.

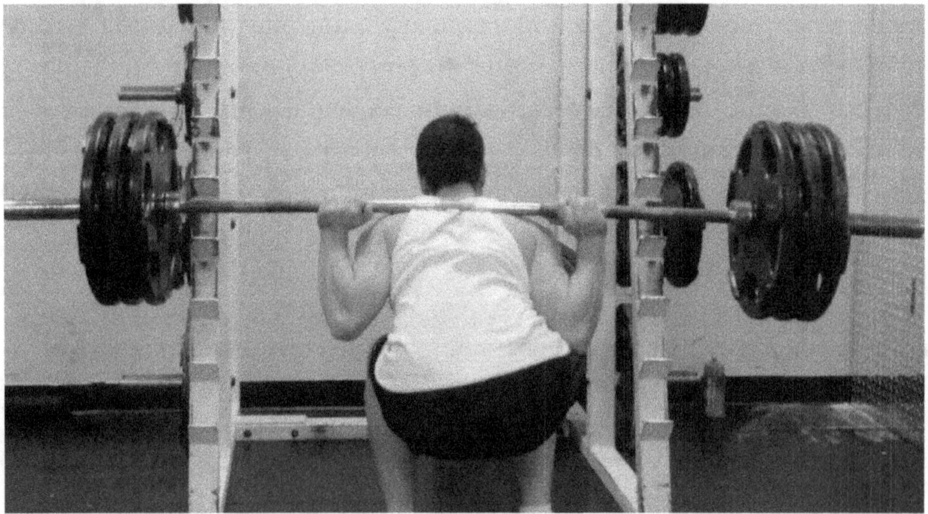

Since you all probably loved my ass shots in the deadlift section, here's another one.

It is in this squatting that the two main risks for injury occur. Should the trainee not squat low enough, he will be bearing that weight on his knees, rather than the muscles of his legs and glutes, and this can lead to nagging injury outside the gym.

And in the "Ass to grass" squat, a trainee that doesn't keep his back and hips tight can risk having lower back movement colloquially known as "buttwink" (in actuality a forward tilting of the pelvis at the bottom of the squat), and this can also lead to lower back and hip injury. If you want to learn posture exercises that will give you the hip flexibility to avoid buttwink, might I recommend purchasing my first (And still most popular at the time of this writing) book *The Oriental's Guide to Sex, Strength, and Satisfaction.*

Once you have gone sufficiently low, the actual lift begins. Push hard through the ground (again I recommend doing this barefoot if you can) and straighten out the legs, while keeping your body straight as it should be. Once you're finished, walk forward and ease the bar onto the rack.

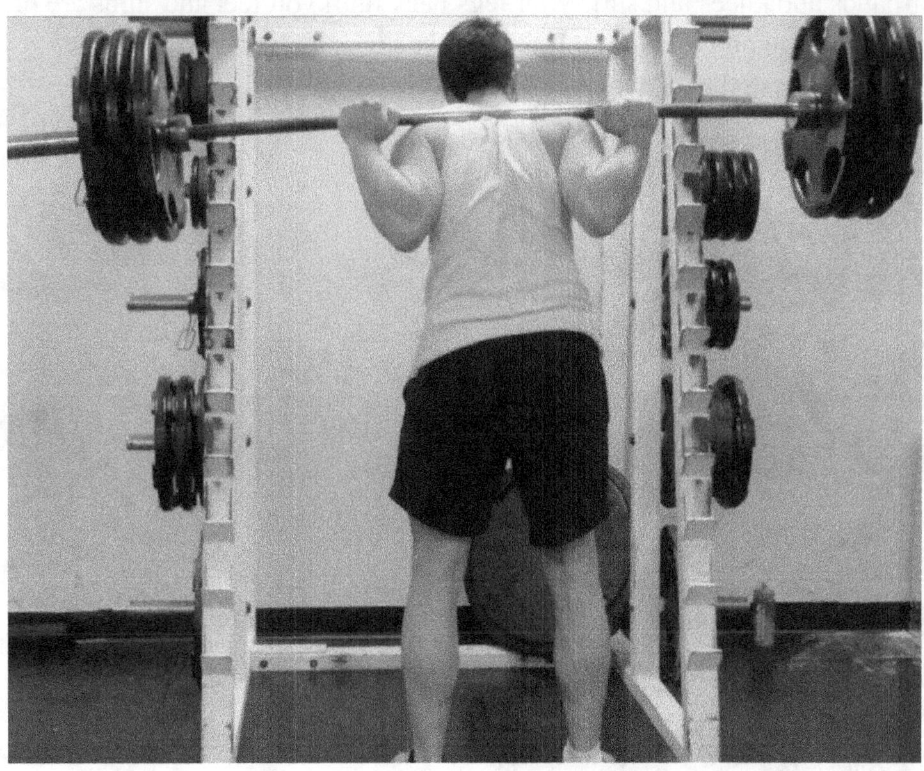

And with that, you know the four main lifts. There are certainly other lifts worth doing, particularly the olympic lifts, but these four will always serve you well, and in doing these lifts, I will hopefully have started your interest in physical culture.

<u>CALISTHENICS</u>

Calisthenics roughly translate to "beautiful body" from ancient Greek, and refer to any exercise that is done against *bodyweight* resistance (as opposed to weighted resistance). To increase the difficulty of these, you have to progress to more difficult variations within a calisthenic "series".

Rather than try to explain, I feel it is much easier just to show you by going through the series. We will begin with the...

PUSHUP

You're probably familiar with this to some extent, and you can likely skip a few steps. More to the point, you probably already know---in theory---the elite step of the push-up series: The one handed pushup! However, in your quest to master the one-handed pushup, remember two things:

A) all calisthenics are done relatively slowly and controlled, with proper form being upheld.

B) And for pushups specifically, you lower yourself until your nose or chin (whichever you prefer) touches the ground.

1) The knee pushup. Most of you will likely not need to do this but I include ot for the sake of completion. Get on your hands and knees and slide your legs back until you feet and shins are off the ground, and you are only resting on your knees. Using the knees as a pivot, do a pushup. Once you can 10 of these, move on to the next step.

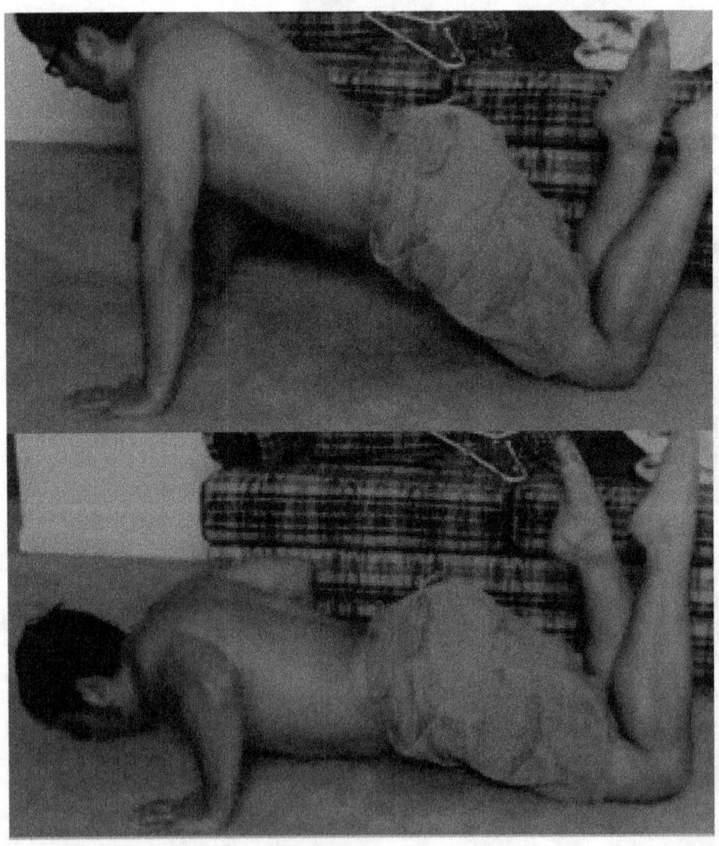

2) The standard you remember from gym class. Keeping the back straight and the hips and buttocks down, bend at the arms and lower your nose to the ground, then push up. Do that 10 times, and move on.

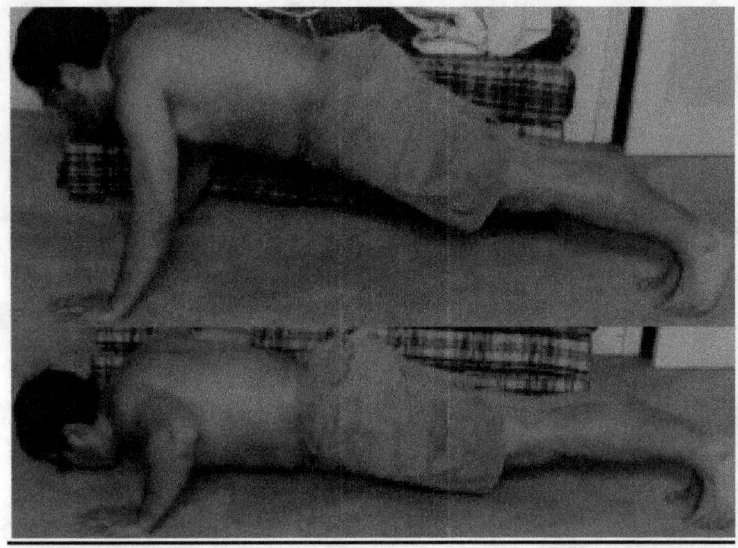

3) the diamond pushup: The hands are brought next to each other forming a diamond shape, and then the pushup is done as usual. If you find these difficult, you can gradually bring your hands closer together. In other words, from the standard pushup, move your hands a couple of inches closer, and then next time another couple of inches closer, etc. until you get to the true diamond form. Once you feel enough of the Illuminati power to complete 10 of these, move on.

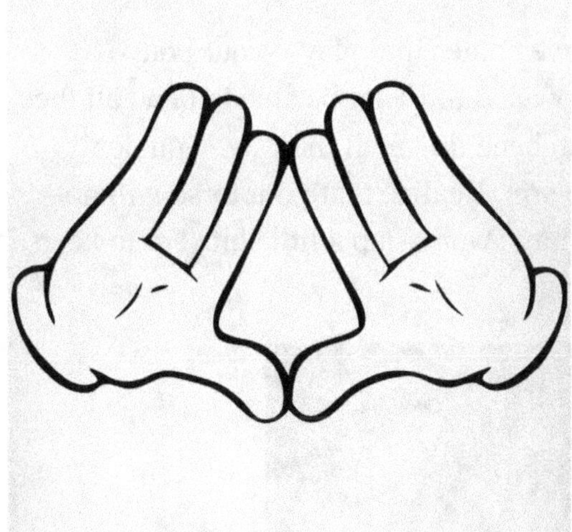

4) "one and a half" hand pushups. Put your hand on a basketball, or something the same size as a basketball (I stacked three books in the picture), and do a pushup. This handicaps the hand that is resting on the object, forcing the other hand to work harder. Do this for both hands. Once you can do 10 with each hand, move on.

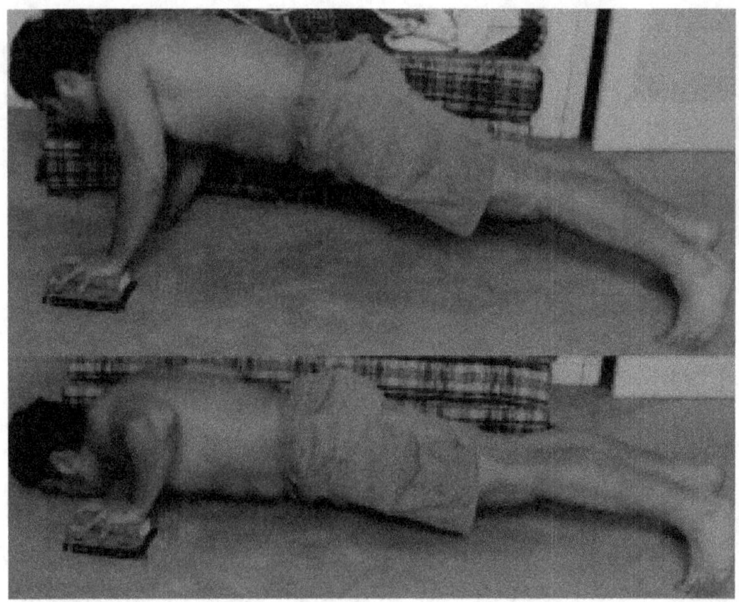

5) Half one-handed pushups, in contrast to the one and a half hand pushup. This is, as the name implies, doing a one-handed pushup, but only going halfway down. Get in a one-handed push-up stance: spread the legs to shoulder width, put the resting hand behind the back, and balance on the other hand (keep the hips down of course). Then bend at the elbow, go as low as you can go, then push up.

This exercise is where the talk of the nervous system above comes into play—your body is simply not used to moving in this way, and you will almost certainly not be able to bend all the way down. Do this exercise with both hands until you can bend down all the way. You don't need to push up, just bend down all the way with the one arm. Realize that your torso will not touch the floor as in the standard pushup, and your hips may "worm" up a little bit. Try to keep the latter to a minimum.

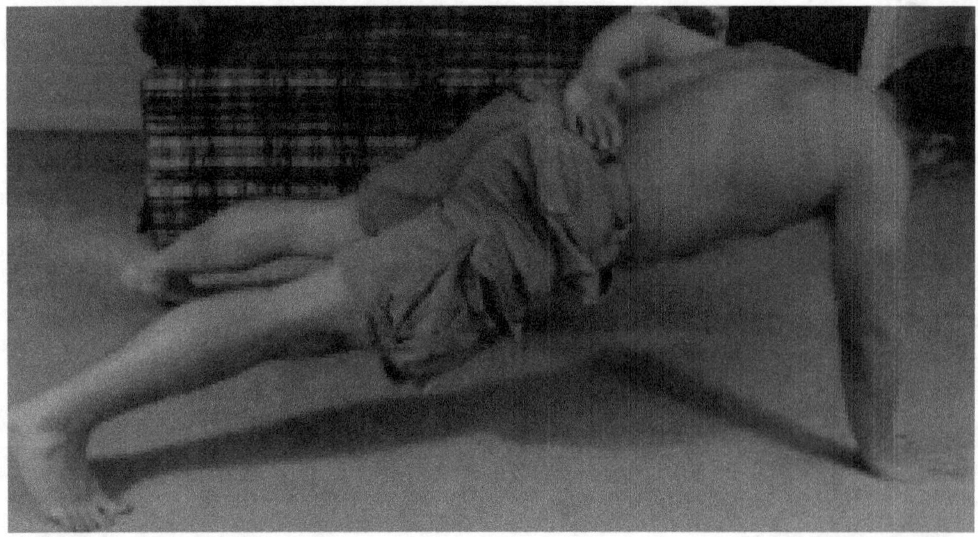

6) Supported one-handed pushups, which are a bit unusual: It's similar to the one and a half hand pushup, but with the supported arm being fully extended—put the supported hand on the basketball (it has to be a ball this time), and roll it out so the arm is extended. Then do a pushup, rolling the ball to your wrist and forearm. The key is not to bend the supported arm. When you can do this 10 times with both arms, you are ready to try the true one-handed pushup.

7) The one handed pushup. As you might assume, the form is identical to the half one handed pushup: you just bend all the way down, touch your chin or nose to the ground, and bend all the way up. You want to avoid contorting your back or hips (pain will tell you when you're doing this).

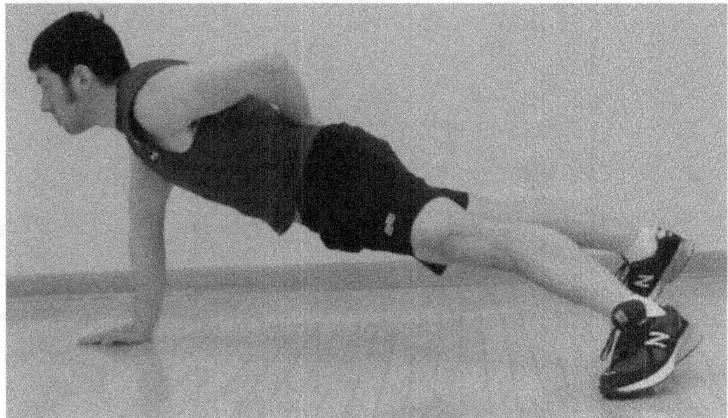

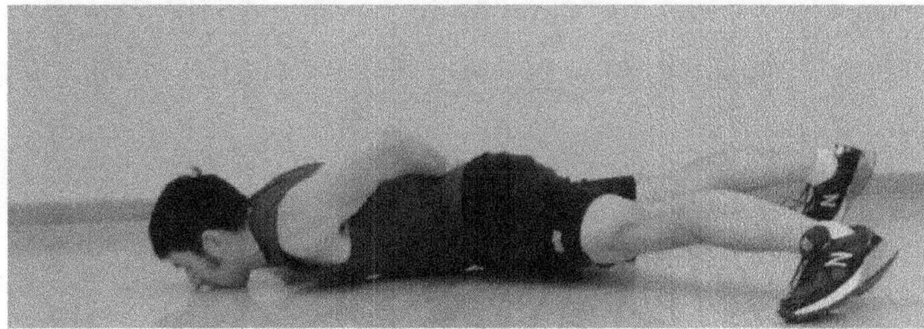

This exact pattern of progressions also works with fingertip pushups, which I have trained to a one handed variation:

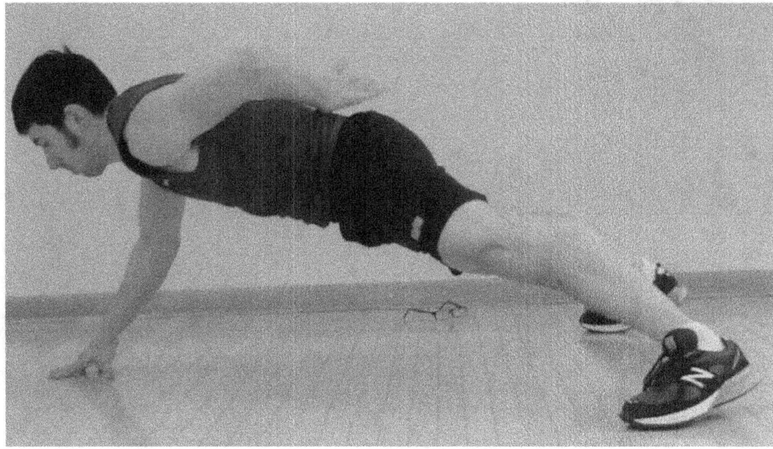

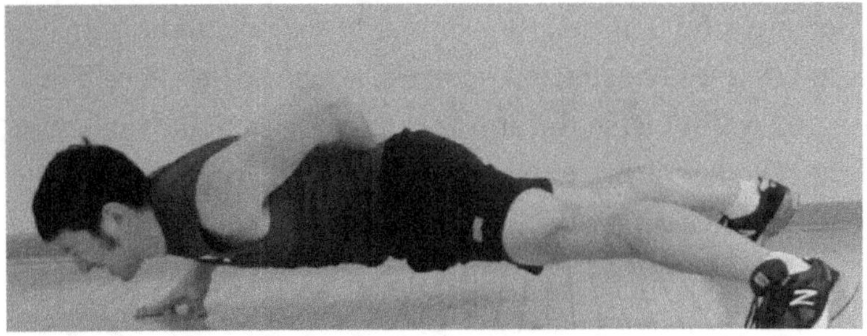

And the same general idea of gradually increasing to progressively harder variations a little bit at a time applies to all calisthenics in general—in effect, it is the bodyweight equivalent of adding weight to the bar.

2) The Squat Series

Training the leg muscles is a necessity for anybody who wants to do any sort of physical endeavor. Simply put, you're going to be standing on your legs throughout whatever sport it is you're playing, and stronger legs means you're going to run faster and jump higher. Learn how to work out those legs!

1) The standard squat. Place your feet shoulder width, and have the feet pointing straight ahead or slightly splayed out. You absolutely do not want your toes to be point inward, as this will cause your knees to knock inward, which can cause stress to your connective tissues. It is important to note that if your ankles or knees hurt when just standing in preparation for a squat, stop immediately and reposition your feet. As this is the same position that the barbell squat is done in, fixing form is imperative before weights are added.

From here, keep the back straight and bend down until your hamstrings touch your calves and you have gone "Ass to grass."

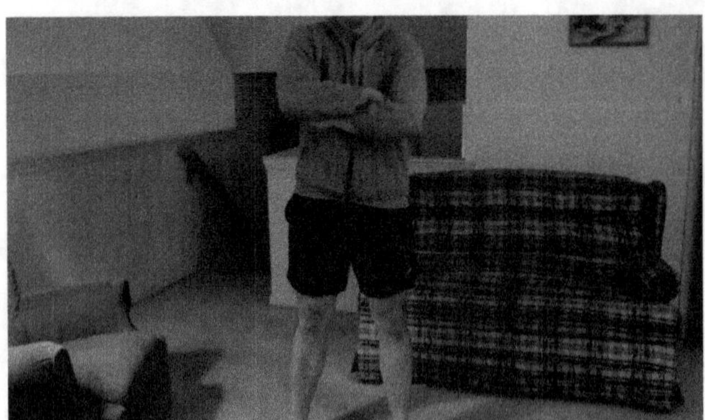

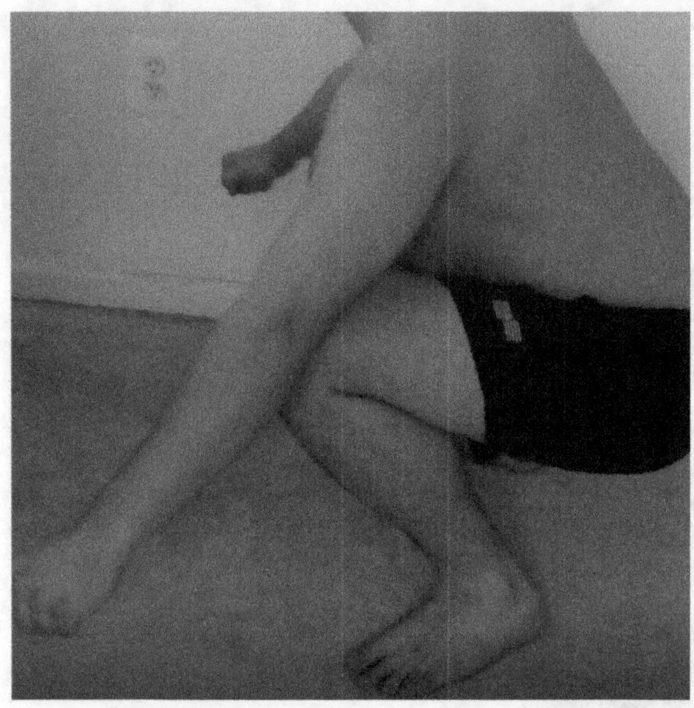

Yes, the standing and kneeling pictures were taken at different times...and days...and months.

Keeping the head up and looking straight ahead helps me keep my torso fixed. Do ten and move on.

2) The heels-together squat, sometimes called the diamond squat akin to the diamond pushup: put the heels together, keep the back straight, and bend ass to grass like the regular squat. This does not really require any more muscular exertion than the regular deep knee bend, but the close proximity of the feet will force you to be off balance, and your body will be forced to compensate. And of course a minor drawback is that doing this exercise will make you look like a pouting emo teenager, but that is a necessary sacrifice. Once again, do ten of these.

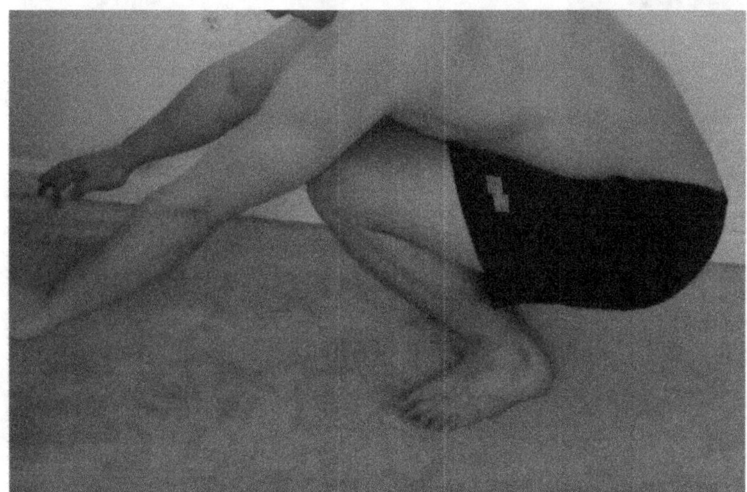

3) The one and a half leg squat. Similar to the one-armed pushup, the next step will also require a basketball or something of similar size (or the wall as I am using). The one-and-a-half leg squat will prepare the body for unilateral movements. Kick one leg out in the air, as pictured

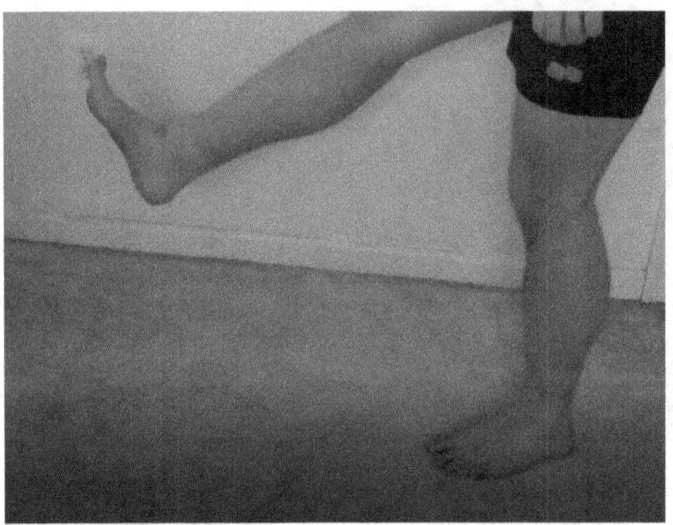

Then bend the other leg until you are ass to grass and the leg is sticking out and straight, with the opposite hand resting on the object (ie: left foot works with the right hand, and vice versa). Positions vary here: Some advocate a flat foot and the leg held in the air as the proper position, while I personally say it's okay to squat on the ball of the foot and have the extended leg touching the floor, as below

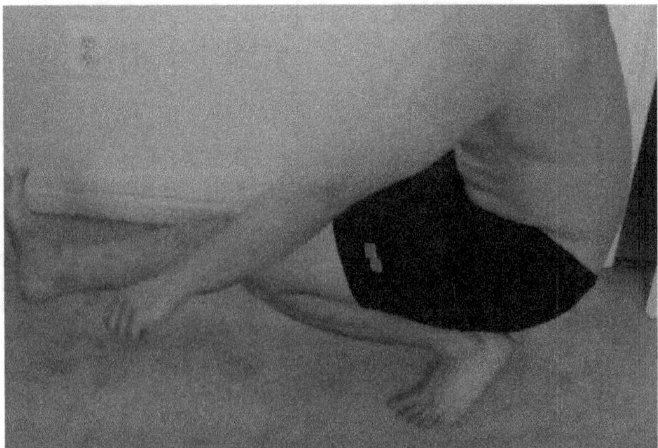

If you choose to have the leg touching the floor, make sure that it is fully extended and only your heel touches the ground-otherwise that foot will assist the lift, and thus take pressure off the squatting leg. Do this for both legs.

Once you can do ten of those, do half pistols-squat down about halfway and then come up. When you can go down all the way (not necessarily coming up), with both legs, move on to the next step.

4) The pistol squat. This is done with the same form as the half pistol. Squat down all the way with one leg extended fully. You will probably have to start out by resting your hand on the floor—as before, do opposite hands and feet. Gradually take your hands off the floor. Perhaps you can embrace your inner cossack and cross your arms over your chest?

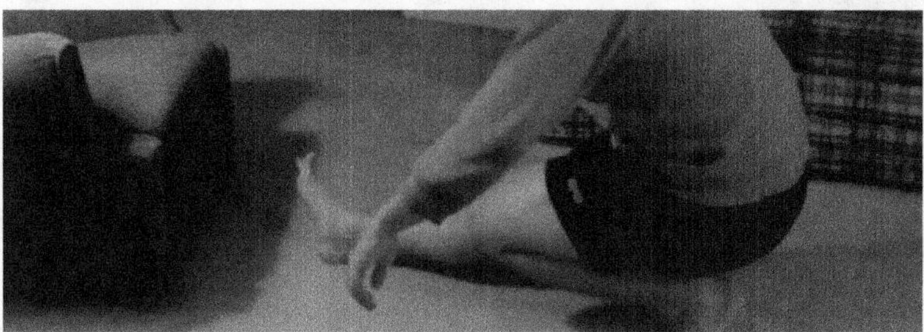

3) The Bridge

You just might be familiar with this one, as some Asian traditions consider the bridge to be the king of exercises. Whether or not those mystical traditions are true, I think you should be interested in an exercise that can heal spinal pain, rejuvenate vertebral discs, add definition and size to muscles most people don't even know exist, tone the arms and legs, strengthen the toes and ankles, expand lung capacity, and promote circulation.

A proper bridge has 4 components: 1) Arms and legs as straight as possible, 2) Arch in the back, 3) Head tilted back in a relaxed position, and 4) Breathing is natural and deep.

To start your bridging education, we will start with...

1) The Short Bridge. Lay down, cross your arms over your chest, and then push the legs and hips up without moving the arms. When you can hold this position for 10 seconds, move on.

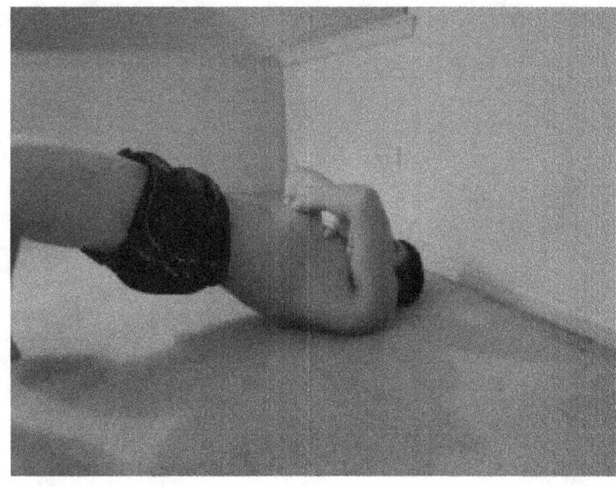

2) The Half Bridge. Get in the bridge position, then roll a basketball or soccer ball under your lumbar vertebrae. Then push off the ground just like the true bridge, but it's easier because you don't have to lift off all the way from the floor. Once this is mastered, attempt the static bridge

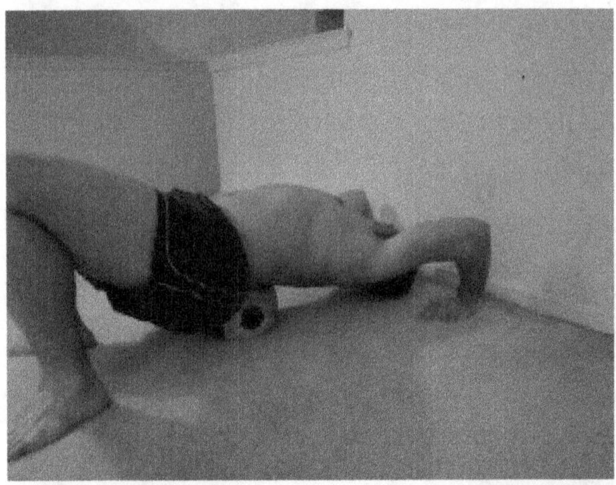

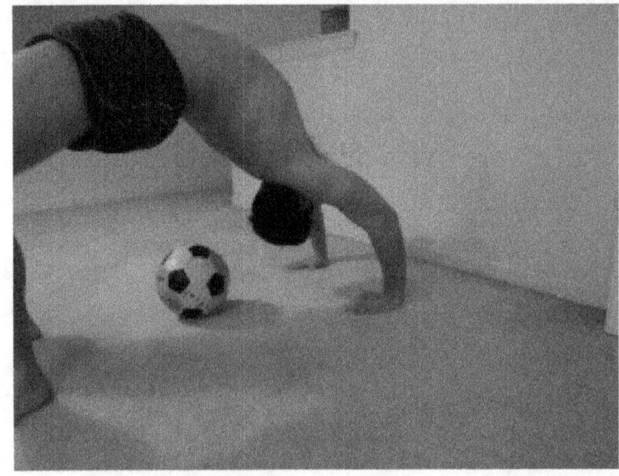

3) The static bridge. Lay down on the floor on your back. Put your feet flat with your knees up. Put your hands flat, palms down, near your temples. Now, simultaneously thrust the hips up as you push down on the floor with your hands and feet. Allow your head to go back between your shoulders. Also note that my bridge fulfills all four components listed above.

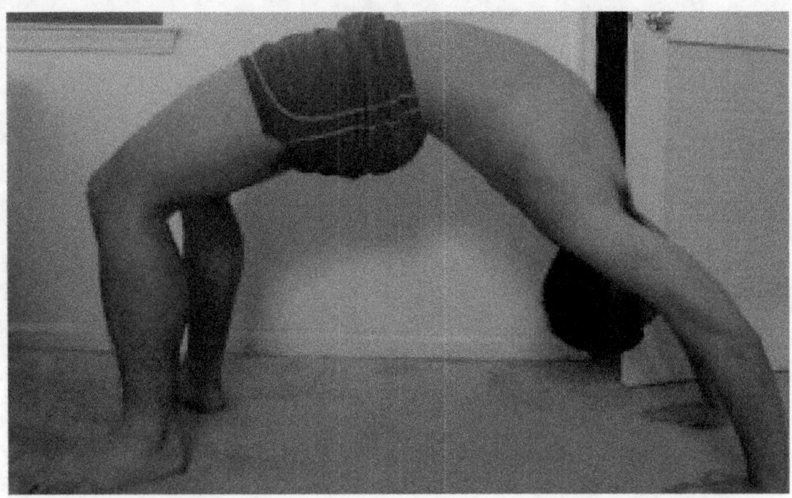

4) The downward wall walk bridge. Now that we have mastered static bridges, we can begin learning active bridges. Stand with your back to a wall, and bend back until your hands touch the wall (palms down, naturally). Then "walk" down the wall on your hands, slowly bending the legs and occasionally stepping forward if needed. If you can't walk down all the way, go down as far as you can, then stop. Do not twist the back, keep it oriented properly.

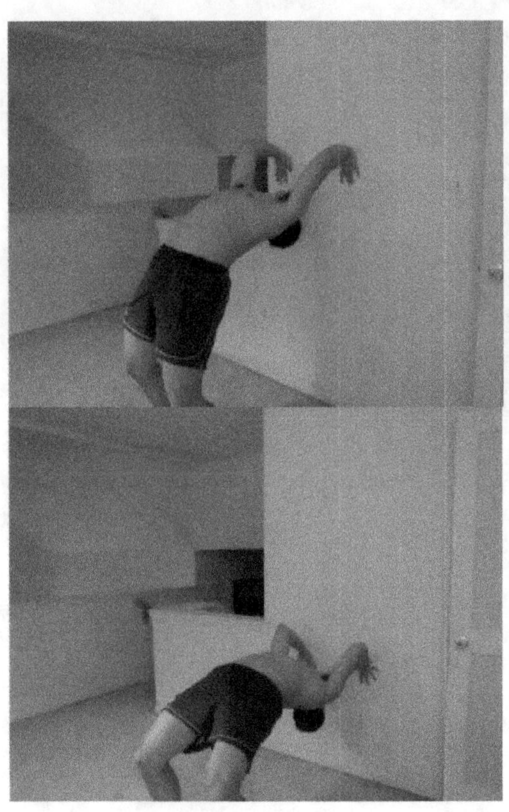

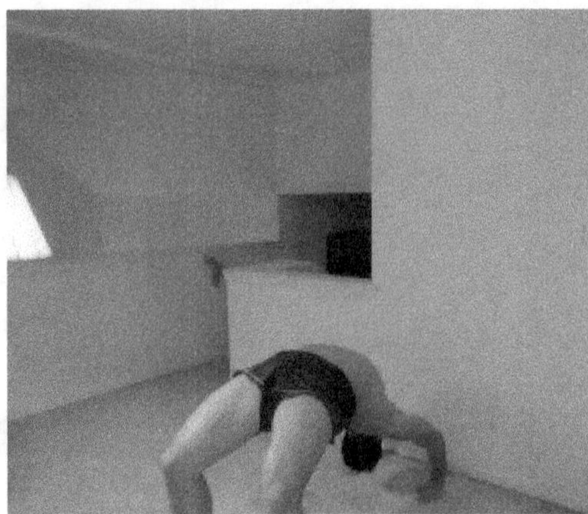

And then attempt to walk back up the wall. When you can do both, without unnatural torsion of the back, move on.

5) The back bend bridge. This is an active bridge without the wall-stand up, put your hands on your hips and your feet shoulder width apart. Get on the balls of your feet, thrust the hips forward, and bend back, until you see the floor behind you. Continue bending and place your hands on the floor. Land gently.

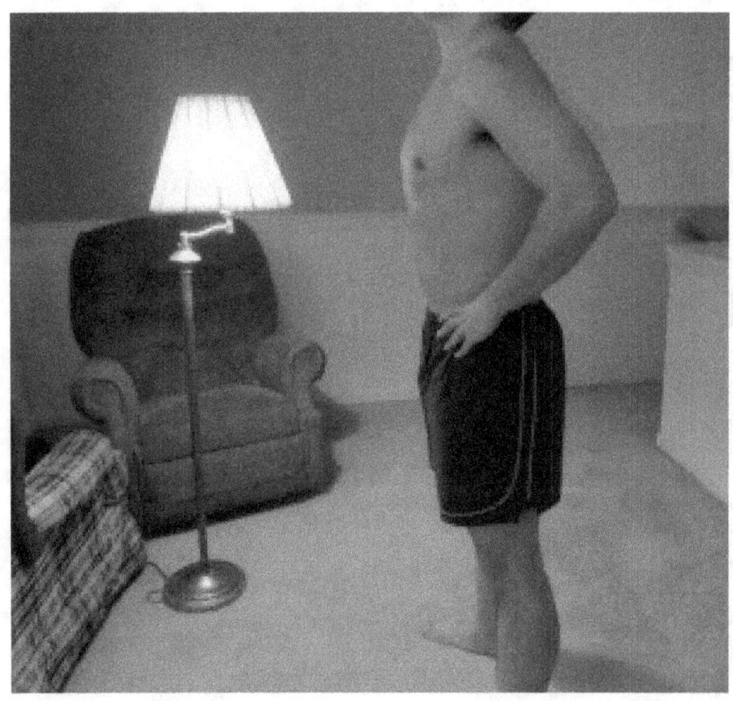

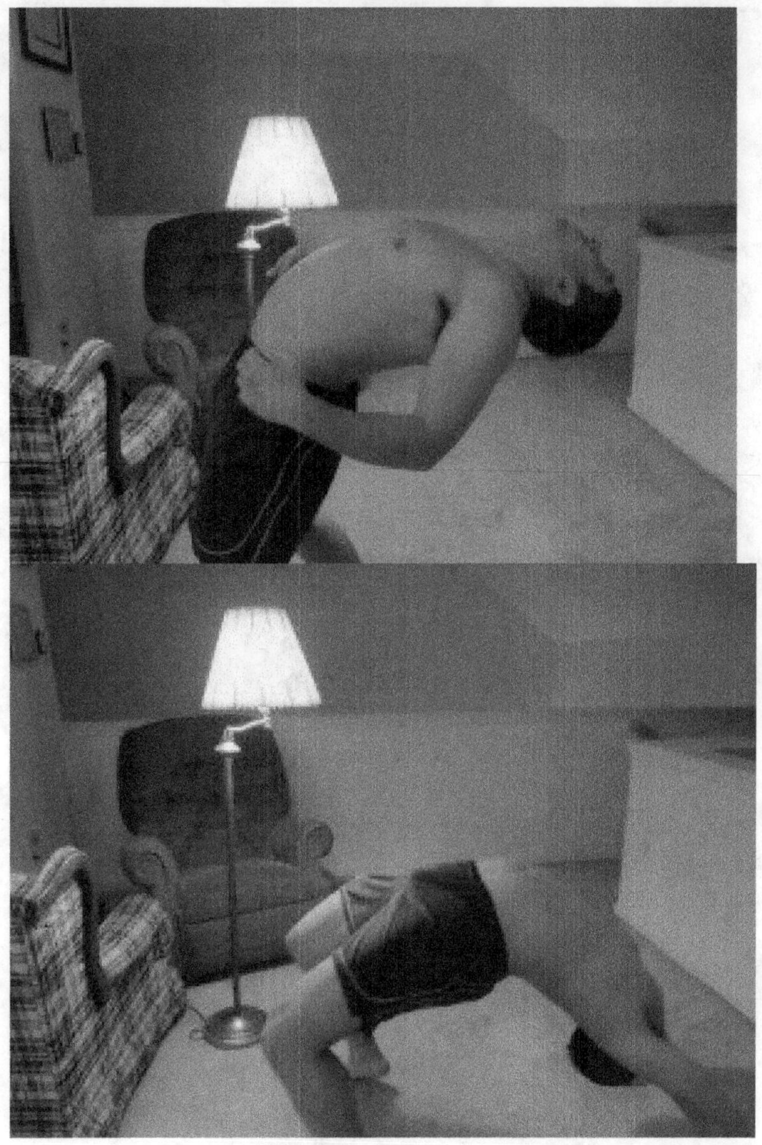

6) The stand-to-stand bridge. First do the back bend bridge, then press down hard with both your hands and the balls of your feet, shift the weight forward, and stand yourself up. It's kind of hard to describe, but it is a highly distinctive feeling. Again, avoid twisting the torso.

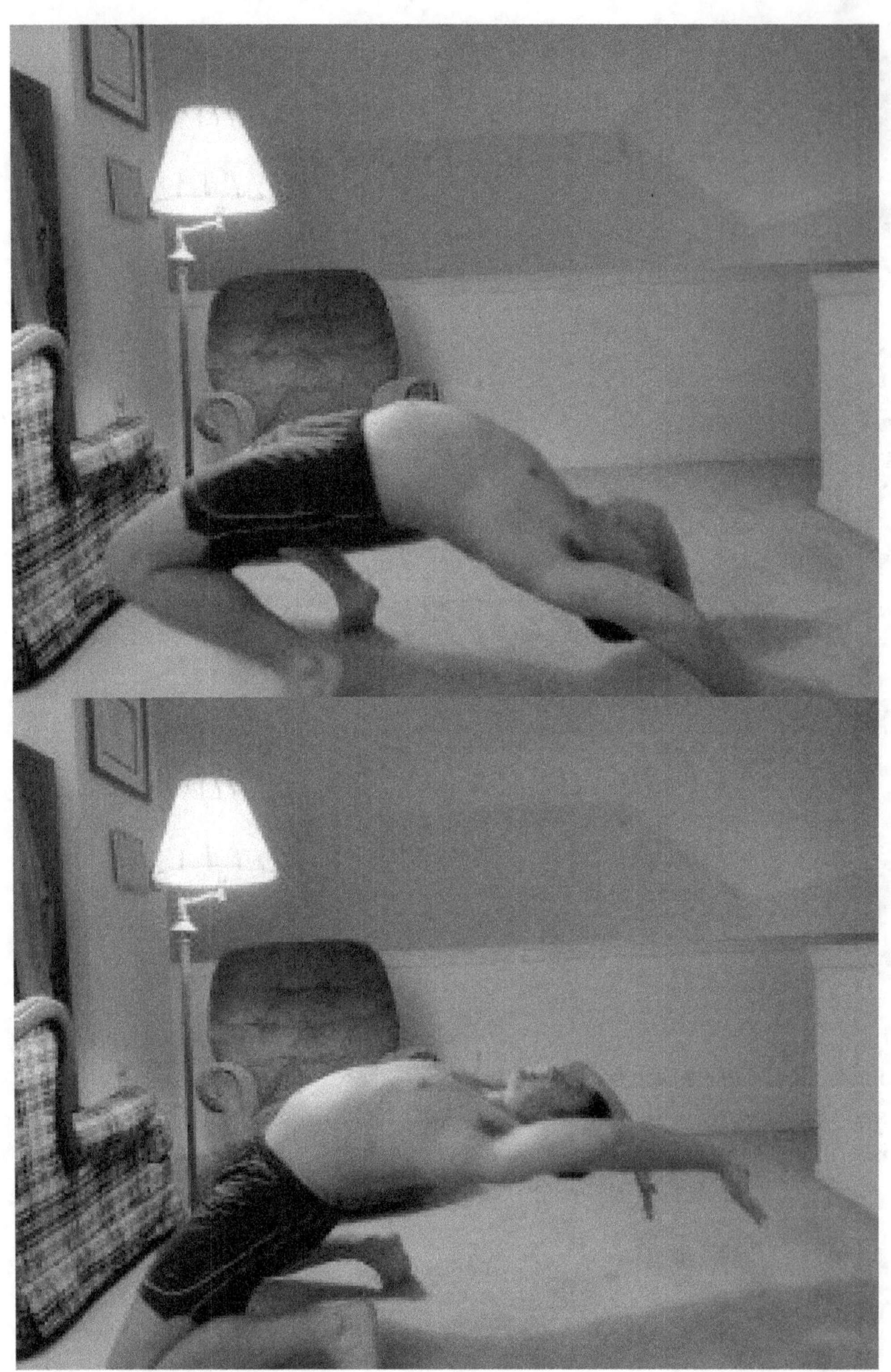

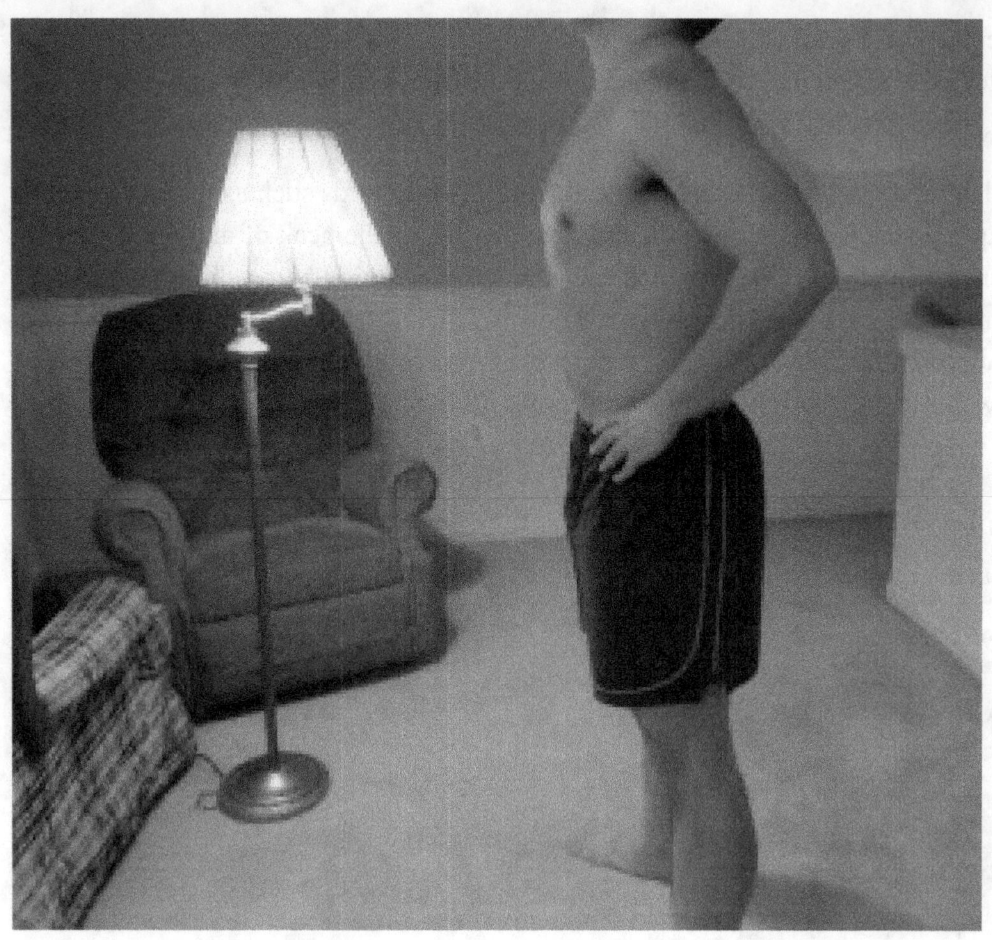

4) The Leg Raise Progression

The hanging leg raise series is a series of exercises that force the abdomen to powerfully
contract. The first of these is the hanging knee raise: Simply grab a hold of a pull up bar, keep
your torso and head upright, and raise your knees together as high as they can go

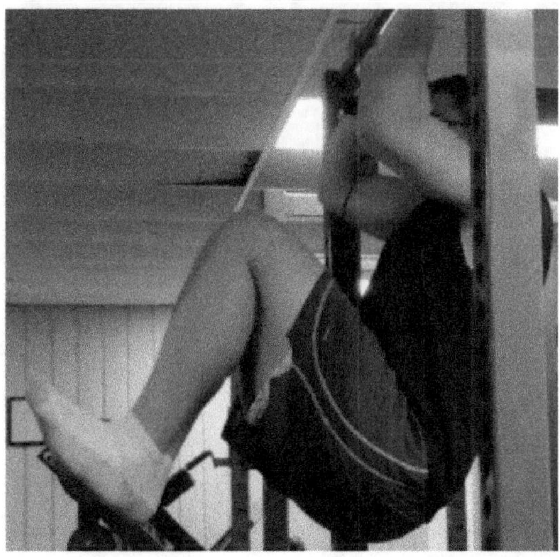

From there, the steps involve gradually extending the legs out each session, a couple of inches at a time, until your legs can swing out fully extended from the hips. But why stop there? Why not lift the legs higher, while keeping the torso in the same position (a move known as the V-Lift)?

Once the hanging leg raise is mastered, you can begin doing static holds such as the L-Sit and VSit for time: Simply do the leg raise or v-lift, and hold the legs at the peak of motion. This exercise can be done on the floor or hanging, with the hanging variation being slightly easier. It is worth noting that the US Men's Olympic Gymnastics team requires a minimum of 60 seconds held for either the floor or hanging L-Sit, and a world-class men's gymnast has core strength any physical culturist would envy (for information's sake, my all time best is 30 seconds).

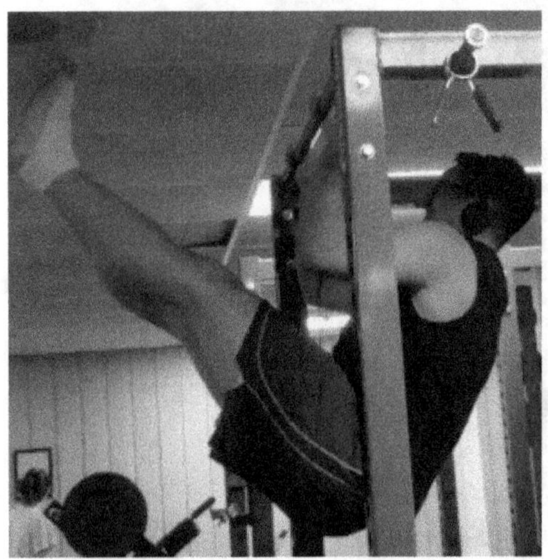

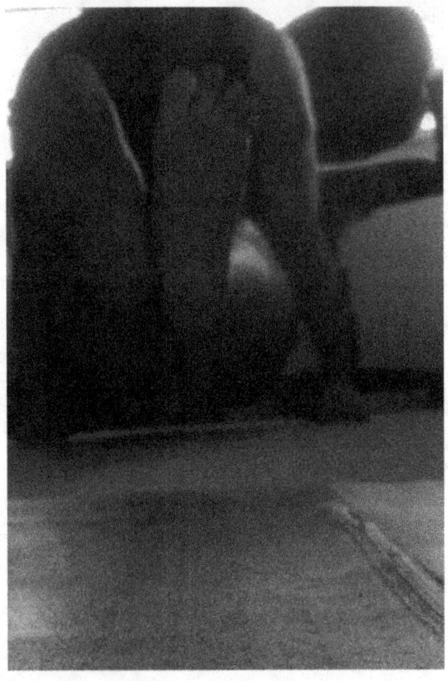

5) The Handstand Push-up series

Unlike the other exercises, you likely have no experience with this, and thus it won't progress as quickly as the others-and I speak from experience.

Doing a handstand, let alone a handstand pushup, seems a daunting, terrifying task. And...yes, it is for a beginner. Trying to do the technique cold will result in you slamming your sacral vertebrae, your head, or both into the ground---hard.

To begin, realize that it is perfectly okay to do the techniques with your feet on the wall. This will build up the strength and muscular power sufficiently, but if you want to do "free" handstands (ie: off the wall), you will eventually need to train specifically for this. Bear in mind that handstand pushups can be done either free or on the wall, but of course they are much easier on the wall due to having your feet on the wall for balance

1) The Headstand. Before you can even do a static handstand, you must do a headstand. put your head on the ground, get into a "sprinter" position, then kick up, with your feet on the wall and your hands and feet bearing your weight. Train this until you can hold it for 1 minute, and then go to the next step

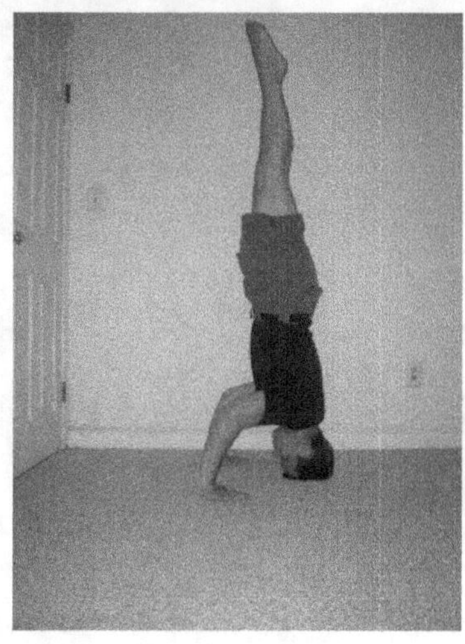

2) The "tuck plank" or the "Crow stand", another static hold: crouch down on the ground with your hands on the floor, tip forward, and bear your weight on your hands as shown below. Hold this for a minute again

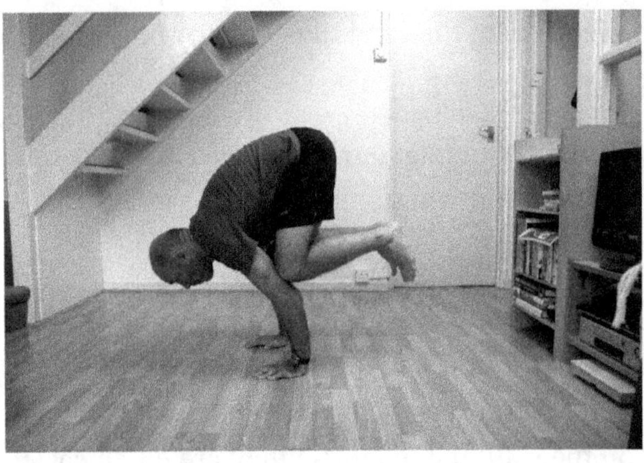

3) the true static handstand. Kick into the handstand on the wall, and hold it for time. After one minute, move on

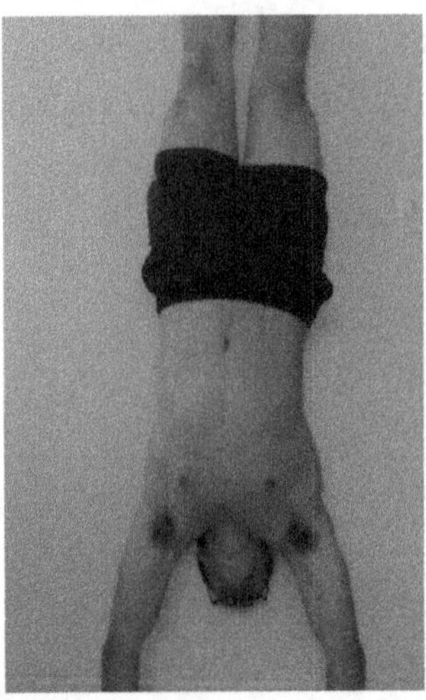

4) Handstand pushups, put your hands shoulder width, descend until your head touches the ground (CONTROL your descent, obviously), and then push back up. If you can't do this, just go halfway, do 10 of those and then try a full descent again. When you can do 10 full handstand push-ups, move on.

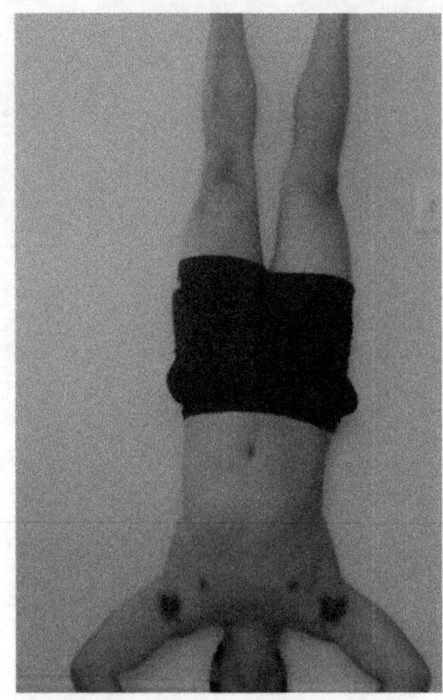

5) Diamond handstand pushups are just like the diamond regular pushups: put your hands together into a diamond, a nd do a pushup. If you can't do a diamond, then gradually bring your hands closer and closer together (ie: from shoulder width, move your hands a couple of inches closer together, and then repeatedly do so until you are doing the diamond)

6) Hand and a half pushups are exactly what you think: one hand on a basketball or stack of books (the latter being easier due to its stability), the other on the floor, and do a push-up. This makes the hand on the floor work harder, as well as training the central nervous system to work unilaterally.

At this point I will admit that gaining weight due to my foot injury has made it difficult to do the other progressions (which were never my strong suit to begin with), but I can still instruct you on how to do it

7) 1/2 one handed pushups are where this series gets really hard: kick into a regular handstand, then remove one hand and put it on the wall. Then do a pushup, going halfway down. This exercise will train the joints and muscles of the shoulder doing the work, as well as the central nervous system. Do 10 with each hand.

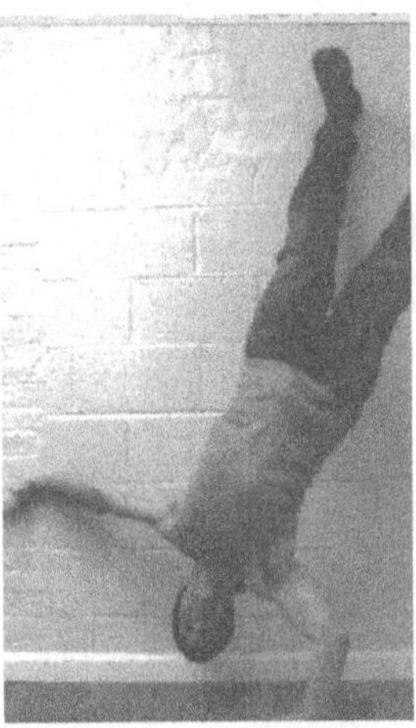

8) The one handed pushup is, to be blunt, extremely difficult, even when using the wall. Get into the same position as step 8, and go all the way down. Do not expect to be able to do more than 1 of these with each hand when starting out (at my best I could only do one with each hand, and I am not at my best)

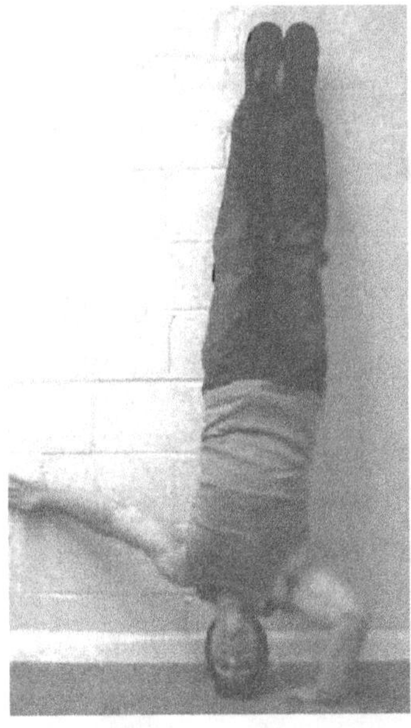

6) The Pull-Up series

The humble pull-up is by far one of the best exercises one can do to develop the upper body, for not only does it develop the size and strength of the latissimus dorsi (the big pulling muscles of the back), it also utilizes the entirety of the upper body as assistance and stabilizers: the forearms, hands, biceps, triceps, shoulders, and the abdomen all get a bit of a workout, as do the small muscles that make up the "rotator cuff." Before I begin discussing the exercise, I must go over the types of grip—more specifically, there are three: anterior grip, posterior grip, and side grip. They differ largely on which muscles of the arm they attack, as all three work the back and torso equally.

The anterior grip has both hands side to side, and the palms facing out. This puts pressure on the triceps, and as such it is usually more difficult for the beginner than the posterior grip pull-up detailed below.

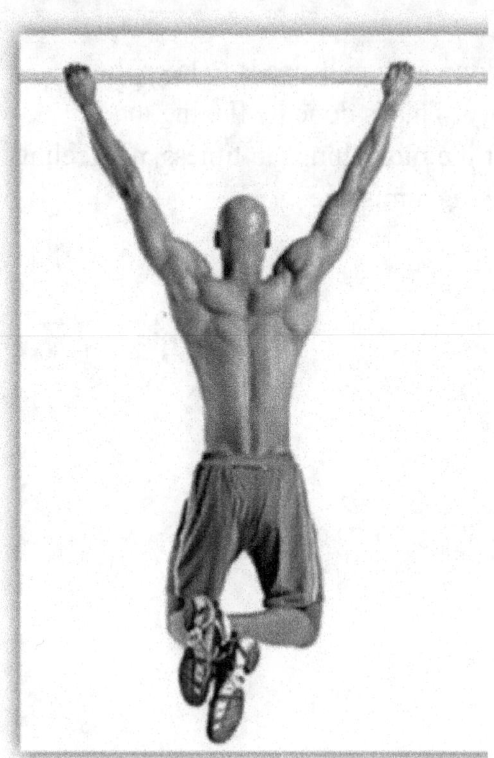

The posterior grip is typically the first one that is achieved by the beginning sportsman. The palms face towards you and it hits the bicep. More accurately, it fully contracts the bicep, hitting the "peak."

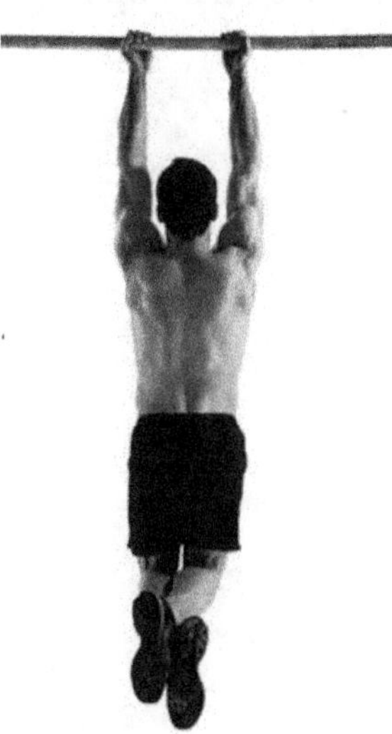

These two grips should be trained by all interested in this exercise, and will serve your needs for functional strength and ability. However, for those seeking aesthetic arms, the side grip can be done, which emphasizes the brachialis and the "short head" of the biceps. Many find this side grip to be more comfortable for one-arm pull-ups as well.

In addition to the grips, a safety precaution that must be done with pull-ups is to keep the shoulders, rotator cuff, and elbows "tight" to prevent injury. This is done by flexing the latissimus dorsi and keeping a slight bend in the elbows. Like most things in fitness, not feeling pain is a sign of doing it right, and pain means you're making a mistake.

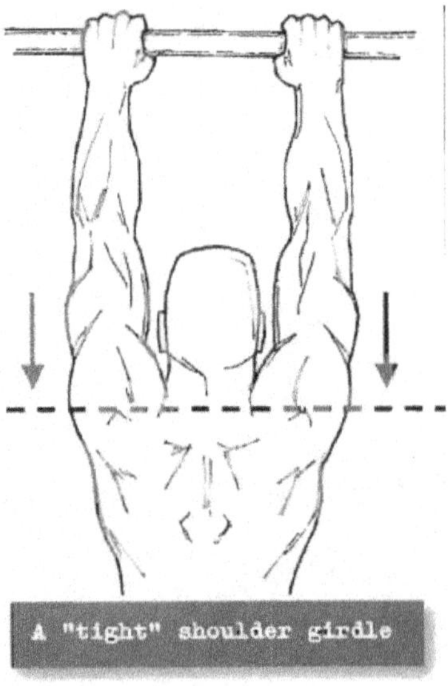

With that knowledge in mind, we can begin the pull-up series:

1) Jack-Knife pulls: these are essentially assisted pullups, where you extend your legs and put them on a chair or another object of similar height, and then pull yourself up. From here on in, the actual pulling maneuver is rather instinctual, and does not need explaining.

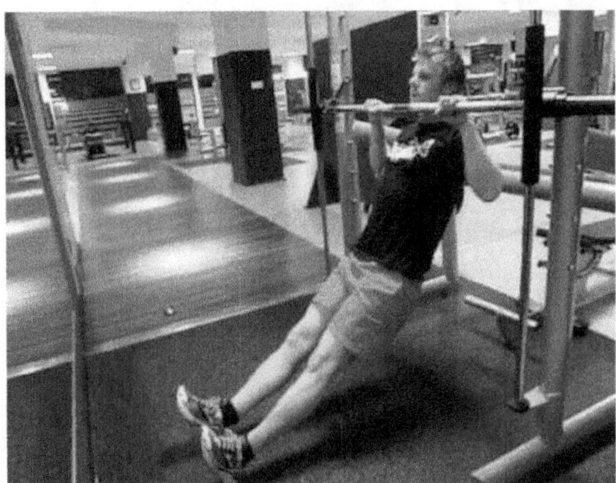

2) Half Pull-ups: These are the first un-assisted maneuver the trainee will perform-jump up into the "flexed arm hang" position your middle school gym teacher let you do as a consolation for failing the pull-up. Then pull yourself up over the bar, and lower yourself into the flexed hang position. And repeat 10 times and go to the next step.

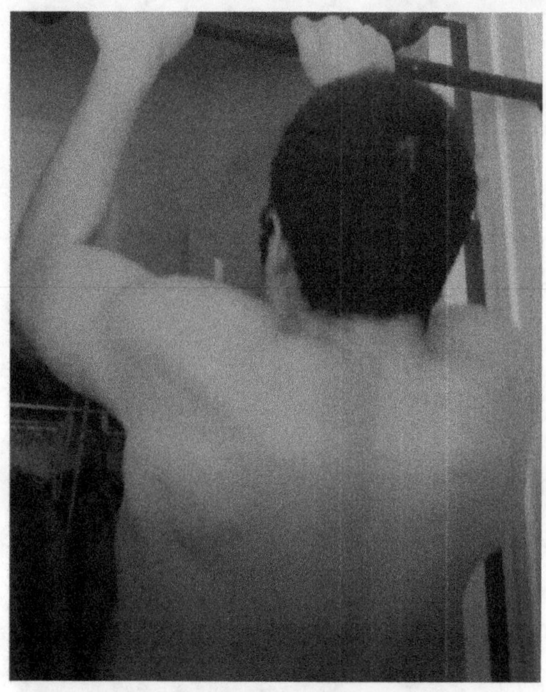

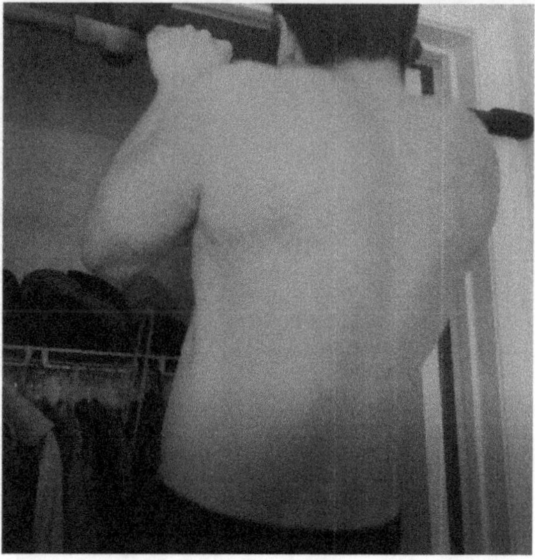

 3) true pull-ups, these are the first exercises in this series that you wouldn't be ashamed to do in public. Just grab the bar, extend your arms to an almost full length (keep a slight kink in your elbows as said above). Then pull until your chin goes over the bar, then lower yourself under control and repeat. I emphasize a controlled lowering, you don't want to just "crash" down and blow out your elbows. Do 10 of these and move on.

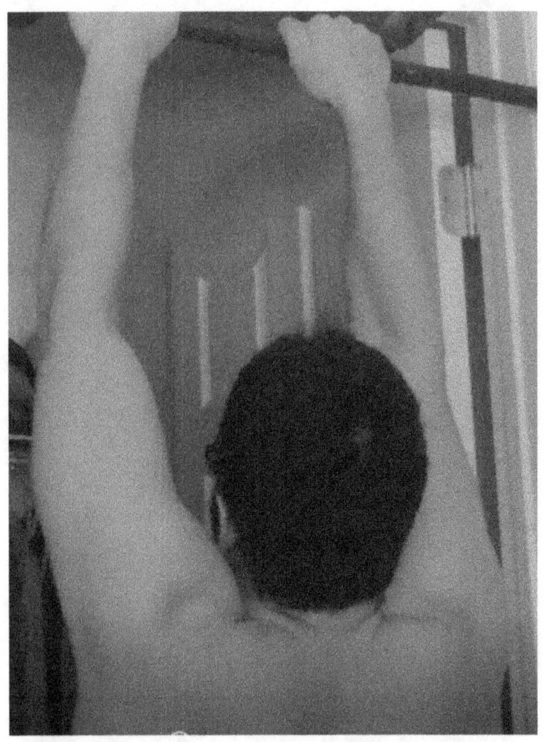

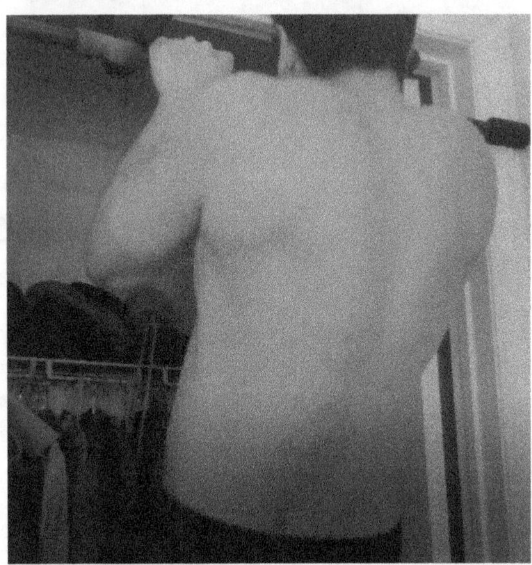

4) Close grip pull-ups. These are, as the name implies, regular pull-ups done with the hands touching each other. This takes pressure off of the lats and puts it onto the shoulders and arms. As such, it is the first step towards one-arm pull-ups.

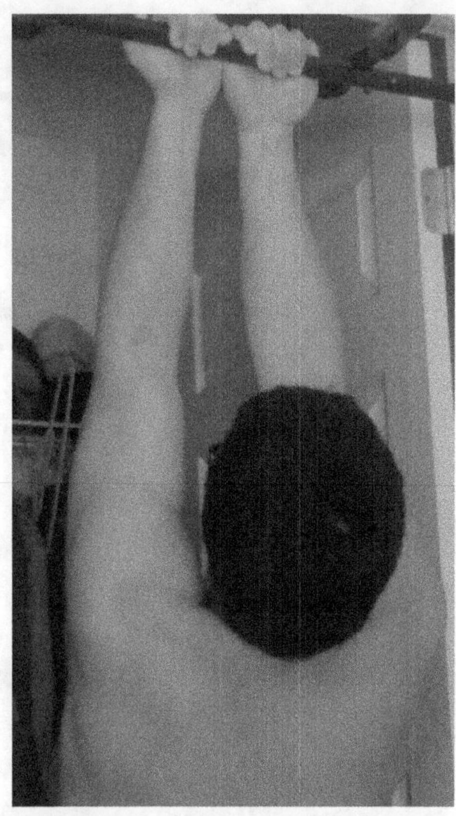

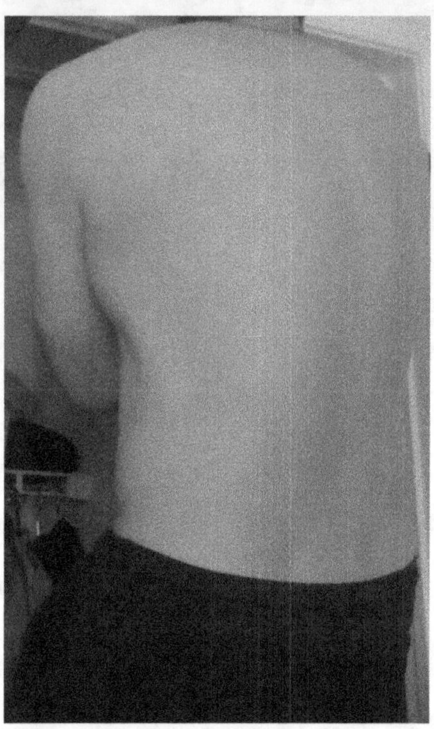

5) Hand-and-a-half pull-ups are something most of us are familiar with, whether it be from Rocky II or seeing some childhood peer doing these, likely referring to them as "one handed pull-ups." Grasp the bar with one hand, and grasp that hand's wrist with the other hand. Then

pull up. This forces the hand on the bar to work much harder than the other. Then switch hands. When you can do 10 of these, move on.

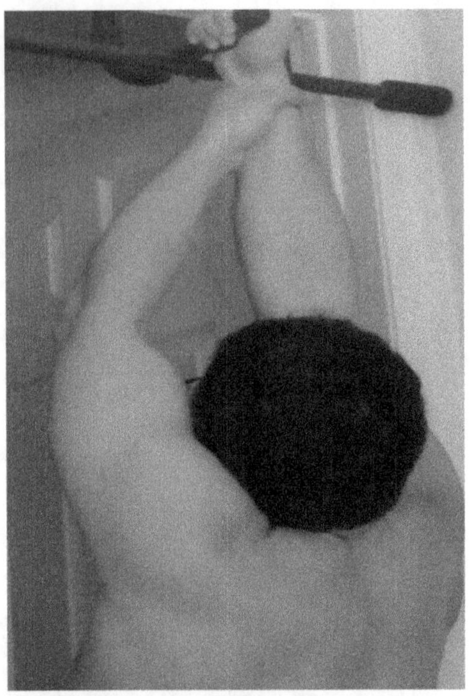

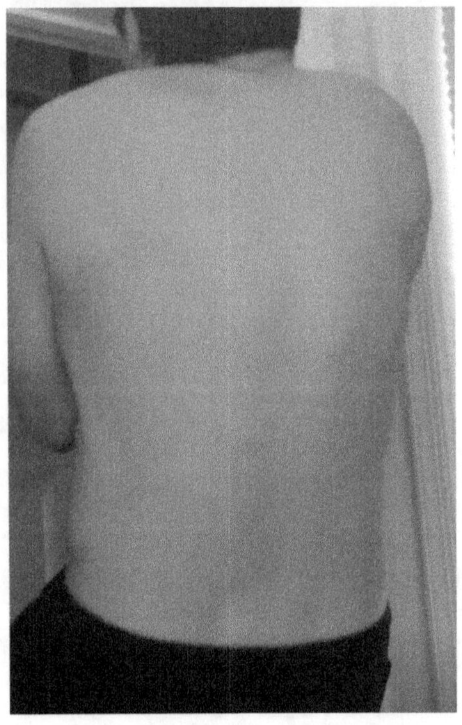

From here, there's not a step, per se, but rather a gradual removal of the fingers gripping the wrist. In other words, do step 7, but release the pinky grip. And then the ring grip, and so forth...

When you're ready, try...

6) The assisted one hand pull-up. This utilizes a towel. Drape it over the bar, and grab it with one hand. Grab the bar with the other hand and pull up from a "dead hang" until the halfway position. Then let go of the towel while simultaneously continuing to pull up and over the bar.

Drop down under control to a dead hang and repeat. Then switch hands. Once you can do 10, take a deep breath and try for the nigh-mythical one-arm pull-up.

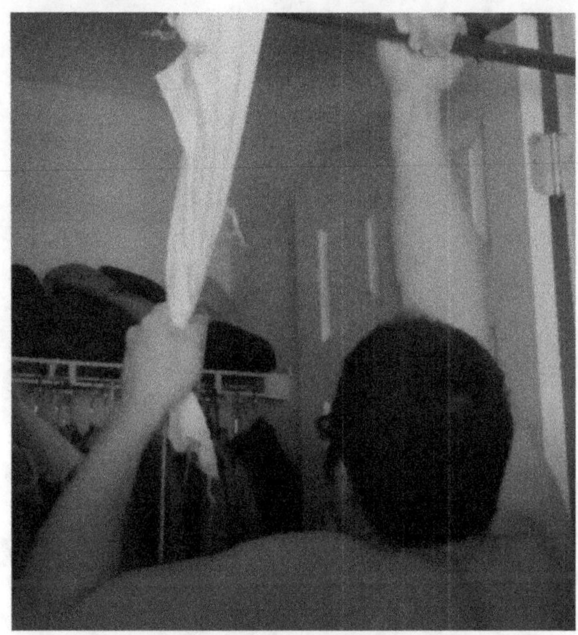

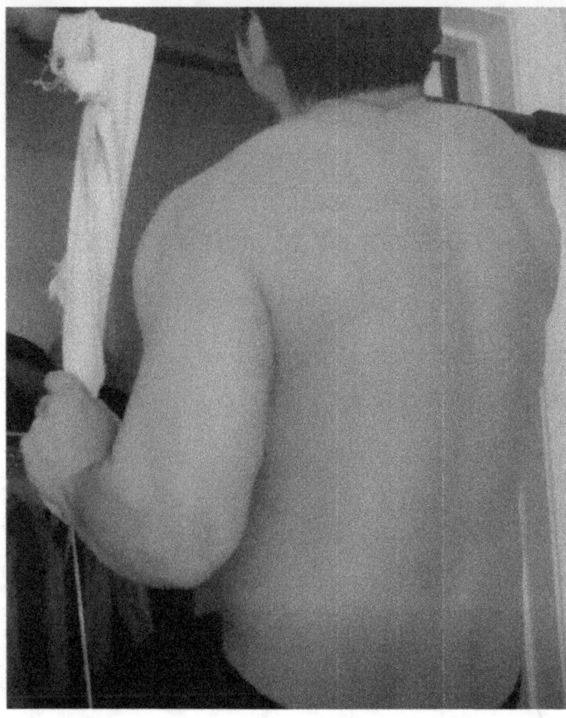

7) The one-hand pull-up. The true one-arm pull up is a feat that's simple in theory, but horrifically difficult in practice. Just grab a bar with one hand and pull with all your might. Once again, my lack of activity due to injury has caused me to put on weight and thus taken away my ability to do this (and even at my best I could just barely do one with only my right hand). Nonetheless these steps will see you through.

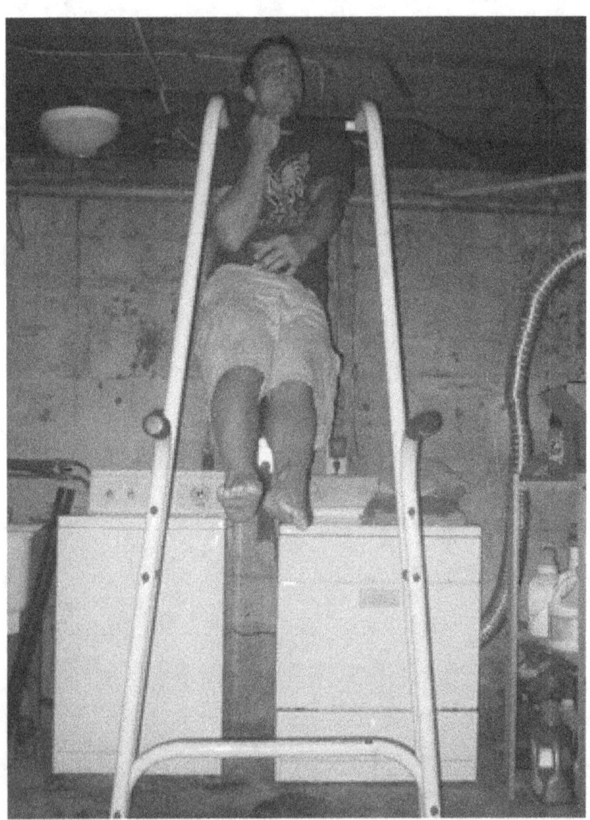

And in mastering those exercises, you will have mastered the basic calisthenic exercises. Should you be interested, you can move into more advanced calisthenics such as the gymnastic fundamentals. Those are beyond the scope of this book, and can be researched by the reader at his will---and arguably the whole purpose of this book is to inculcate a love of fitness in the reader, which you likely will once you see your body changing.

Now, having thoroughly learned how to do resistance exercise, we can begin doing cardio. Remember to alternate exercises on different days, like was previously discussed.

Cardio

What is cardiovascular exercise, and how do we define it? It is any exercise where the primary goal is to get the heart rate up and increase your overall endurance. In other words, it differs from resistance training in which the predominant goal is to build maximal strength and possibly <u>muscular</u> endurance.

Why do you even need cardiovascular endurance at all, you might ask? To answer that question, go find a flight of stairs, preferably one with multiple levels. Once you've done that, run up the stairs as fast as you can.

Did you do it? You're probably gasping for air and clutching feebly at your torso---and <u>that</u> is why you need cardio endurance. Simply put, if you don't have it, you don't have the capacity to do anything: not walk around day to day, not any of the activities you like to do, *nothing*.

And for weight loss, cardio burns more calories in less time than any other exercise form, if done in certain (Strenuous) ways.

Why did I discuss heavy lifting first, then, if cardio is so damn good? Because the two forms of exercise done in conjunction is greater than the sum of the parts. While cardio burns many calories, it does not induce the hormonal changes associated with heavy resistance training and does not produce the same skeletal muscle building results.

Indeed, taking a look at those who do nothing but cardio...

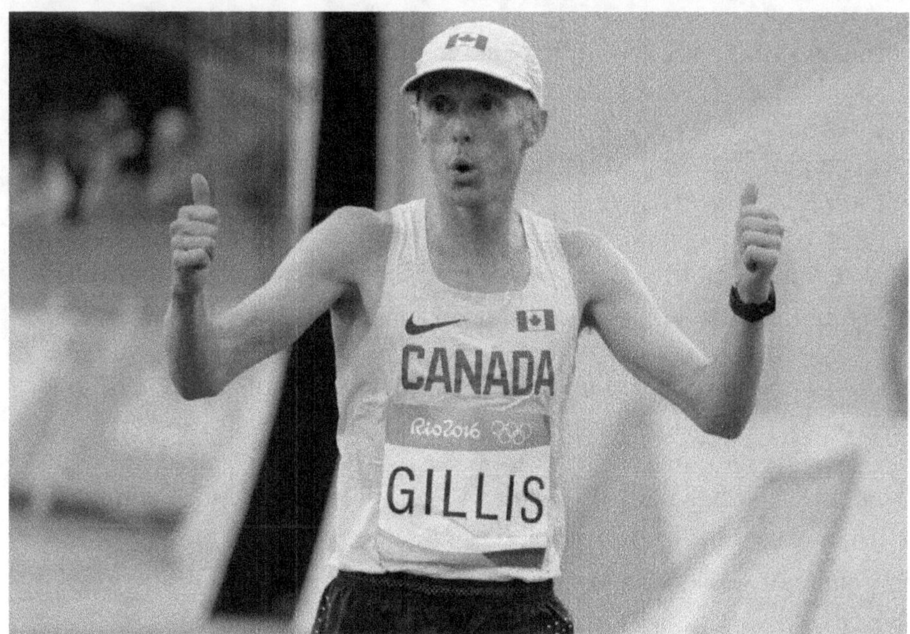

...we can see that they're not exactly Adonises, no? In fact, "Watery" or "emaciated" is the word that springs to mind.

Conversely, however, focusing entirely on strength training isn't so good either:

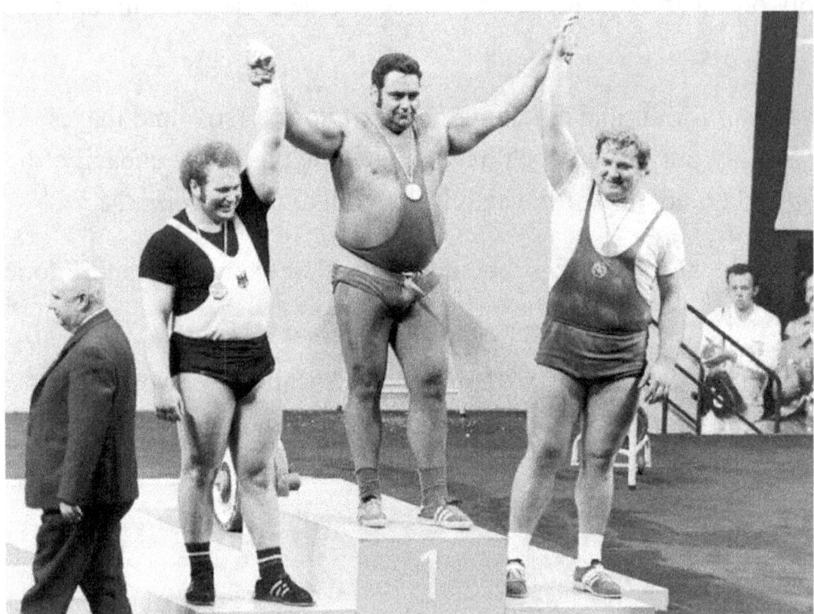

Chaps like these are monstrously strong, but I doubt they could run a mile without dying of a heart attack.

The other reason I discussed weights first, and so intensively, is that compared to resistance training, cardio is almost absurdly simple. To do cardio is simply...to move!

Get out in the world, and move quickly until you get winded, and then keep moving until you reach some pre-determined point that is to your satisfaction (like, say, a mile).

Running, biking, swimming...the possibilities are myriad! You can also run on a treadmill or pedal an exercise bike if you enjoy feeling like a rat in a maze (I don't).

If running is too hard for you, try walking. Walk a mile or two for a few weeks until you feel confident in running a bit. Then walk 75% of the way and run the last 25%, and gradually do more running over another couple of weeks. It's just like the weights, start low and slow and gradually build up.

And that's really all you need to know for cardio---set goals, consistently expand and increase your gogals, and don't do cardio and resistance training on the same day. Cardio is simple, in marked contrast to...

Chapter 4: Dexterity

Dexterity is a somewhat nebulous concept, and indeed I would argue that it is secondary to the other two aspects of fitness we have previously discussed. However, the secondary exercises do wonders in preventing injury and increasing mobility, so why wouldn't you want that?

Some of my male readers might be groaning already, saying that this is predominantly a "woman's goal" of fitness, citing the always-prevalent female desire to "tone" and "lengthen" muscles without adding bulk. And while stretching certainly accomplishes these things, there are many benefits specifically for the masculine man, such as:

Improved posture, increased athletic ability, and increased mental fortitude and tolerance to pain (why else would the *Spetsnaz* force all their recruits to be able to do a "wishbone" split?)

Also, bear in mind that stretching should never be done on the same day of cardio or resistance training. I do it after my martial arts practice, but bear in mind that good, worthwhile stretching is a workout in and of itself.

My dexterity training is part and parcel with my martial arts practice, but for your purposes, I will take them out of their kung fu context and repurpose them for purposes of general flexibility training.

Before we can discuss what stretches to do, we have to learn *how* to stretch---that is to say, the theory behind stretching. This is likely something you have never even heard of, so allow me to explain.

Like most exercise programming worth a damn, the concept of "Relaxing into a stretch" comes from our dear friends the Soviet Union. To explain what relaxing into a stretch is, it's easier to explain how you *shouldn't* stretch, in a direct antithesis to a relaxing stretch.

How Not To Stretch

Many people believe that stretching is a literal act of forcing the muscles and connective tissue to stretch—**avoid this at all costs**! First and foremost, you should never apply any stretching pressure to the connective tissue. They evolved solely to "hold fast" and keep things in one piece, they should never be stretched at all!

The muscles are the anatomical feature that stretches, as they evolved to do. When stretching, your body should always be positioned in a way where the connective tissues are stable and the muscles are moving.

Even when you are positioned properly, no part of stretching should involve the athlete forcing his muscles to stretch, as that risks muscular tearing which is a nagging injury that never truly goes away. This is because the human body has naturally evolved what is referred to as the "anti-stretch reflex" to prevent muscular tearing-stretching the muscles increases in difficulty the farther and deeper the stretch is, and your body responds to this stress with pain. This is a biological sign telling you that if you go further you'll be risking muscle tears, and should normally be a heeded warning.

However, if you want to do advanced stretching (such as that nigh-impossible benchmark of fitness the splits), you will have to find a way to overcome this reflex without hurting yourself. And as luck would have it, there is!

Relax Into Stretching

Reflexes can be overcome with gradual and repeated practice—just ask your friendly neighborhood hooker (er, "nymph of the pave", "beindl", or whatever old-timey synonym for a "soiled dove" you want to use to keep up the "peasant" theme) about how she overcame her gag reflex! Similarly, your anti-stretch reflex that keeps your "joints" (actually your muscles) stiff and immobile can be overcome with a few techniques.

The most basic of these techniques is the one that I have had the best results with (as usual, the simple but difficult answer is usually the correct one), and that is the titular concept of "relaxing into a stretch"—with thanks to Pavel Tsatsouline for naming the concept.

To use this technique, take an easy form of the stretch you want to do: using the splits as an example, you would do a seated groin stretch. Engage the stretch just to the point where you feel tension in the target muscle, and then…sit and wait.

Yes, paradoxically, relaxation is the key to increasing your physical fitness in this context. You are literally going to sit there and wait for your muscles to stop fighting the stretch—in other words, you're going to exhaust your reflex until it stops being reflexive.

This is not something that happens quickly—from my experience, it will take 5-10 minutes per stretch, so it is perfectly acceptable for you to get a book or watch TV while doing this. As a side note, this is literally the only time where it's acceptable to have a visual distraction during exercise, in my opinion.

As you might expect, once your muscles have relaxed and the pain has melted away, you can increase the stretch a little bit more, and hold it for another 10 minutes. Repeat this process until your muscles are in pain and you judge that you can't go any further—this is a personal call that you will have to decide for yourself, as I can't judge when your muscles are demanding you to stop.

This technique can be utilized for any stretch, and in many cases will give you the progress that you so desire. However, there are other methods in the "Relax Into Stretch" family of exercises that can be utilized as well, such as meditation—mentally relaxing will lead to muscular relaxation.

Or you can try "forced relaxation", where you flex the muscle simultaneously while stretching, forcing the muscle to relax.

Just remember to breathe regularly and naturally.

Try it yourself!

ACTUAL STRETCHES

Okay, now we're getting into the actual meat and potatoes of flexibility

The first stretch I would have you learn is one you have probably not seen before, but when combined with the aforementioned bridge, will clear up about 90% of your lower back pain (if you have any): the twist stretch!

Most people seem to not consider upper body flexibility when doing any sort of flexibility training, but that is just as important to train as lower body flexibility (namely for purposes of increased athletic performance, reduction of joint aches and pains, and, in some cases, increased strength). In my opinion, if you're going to do any one stretch for upper body flexibility, that would have to be the seated twist stretch.

How It Works

This stretch involves crossing your legs in a manner that will be discussed below, and twisting the torso while simultaneously locking your arm onto your bent knees. This stretch will hit most of your most prominent upper body muscles—the latissimus dorsi, the triceps, the deltoids, the obliques, the neck, and the pectorals.

In addition to those visible muscles, the twist stretch will work the deep spinal muscles, and even the muscles of the buttocks (the gluteus maximus, medius and minimus) as well.

Many athletes perform the twist stretch, particularly combat athletes such as wrestlers, judokas, and mixed martial artists that need great torso flexibility to escape from holds and pinfalls.

Sounds like something you ought to learn, doesn't it? But how?

As I have happily admitted in the past, and will likely do so again in my writing career, Paul Wade's outstanding *Convict Conditioning* series has taught me this and many other exercises, and I cannot advocate Wade's writing enough. More specifically, the Twist Stretch comes from *Convict Conditioning 2*. The first book deals with the core calisthenic series—push-ups, squats, and the like. I have already gone over these in detail. In contrast, the second book deals with static holds that develop strength and flexibility such as the L-Sit and today's topic.

The Exercises

The first twist stretch is the "Easy twist stretch." Sit down on the floor with your feet extended. Take one foot, and put it "inside" the other leg, resting that foot next to the opposite knee, as shown.

Now, twist your body so the opposite shoulder turns towards the raised kneed (ie: if the left knee is raised, turn the right shoulder, and vice versa). Keep the foot flat on the ground and the knee stationary-just twist the torso. Allow your neck to turn as it naturally wants to turn.

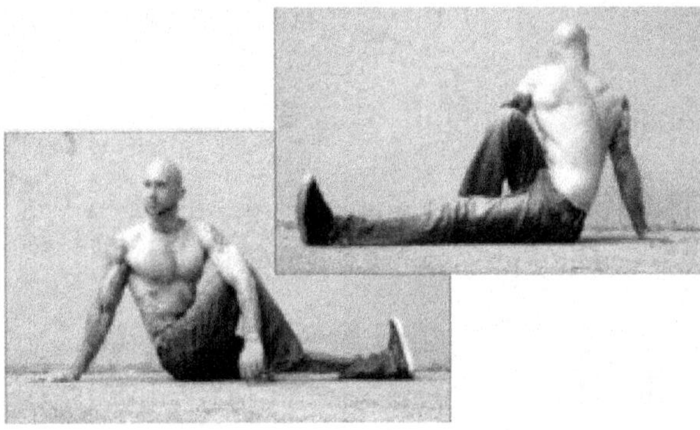

Then, "lock" your torso by placing your elbow against the opposite side of the knee, while holding your body up with the other hand.

You should immediately begin to feel a stretch all around your torso.

Hold the stretch for 10 seconds, for each side. When this is comfortable for you, move on.

Step 2 is the simple twist stretch, which requires a little bit more flexibility. Place one foot over the other leg as shown above. Then, take the foot that is not flat on the ground, bend the leg back and touch the heel of that foot to the opposing buttock (ie: the right heel touches the left buttock).

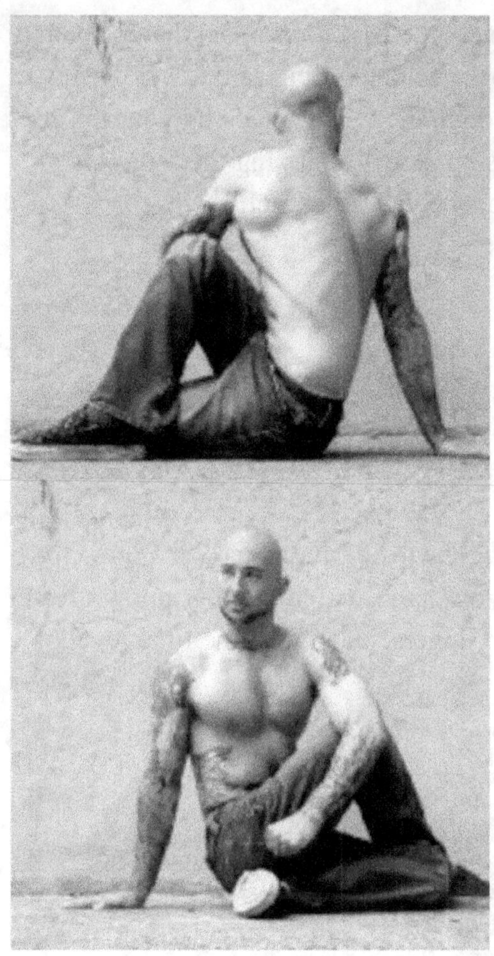

This foot position will be used for all twist stretches from henceforth.

Now, as before, rotate your torso towards the opposite knee (right shoulder to left knee, and vice versa), locking yourself by placing your elbow on the opposite side of the knee, and again supporting your body with the other hand. Hold for 10 seconds, and move on.

Stretch 3 is where things become more difficult. Assume the position from Stretch #2. But this time, you will have to rotate the torso with much more force, as the goal of this stretch is to extend your arm and touch the instep of the foot that is flat on the floor. Your arm won't be able to stretch on its own (and I don't advise you try), you will have to accomplish this with proper torso rotation.

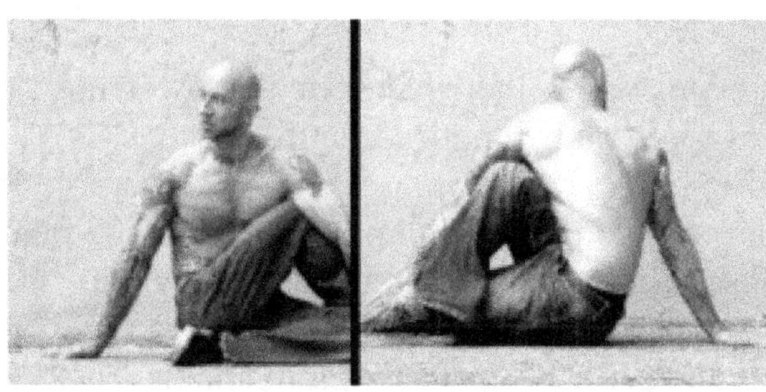

Stretch 4 has the difficulty increase further: Get a hand towel or some other object that is about a foot long. Assume the stretching position, and rotate the torso while holding said towel. Remove the supporting hand from the floor, and flick the towel through the "hole" made by your raised leg (obviously your hand is not extending down to your instep here). Wrapping the "support" hand around your back, grab the other end of the towel. This begins the stretch.

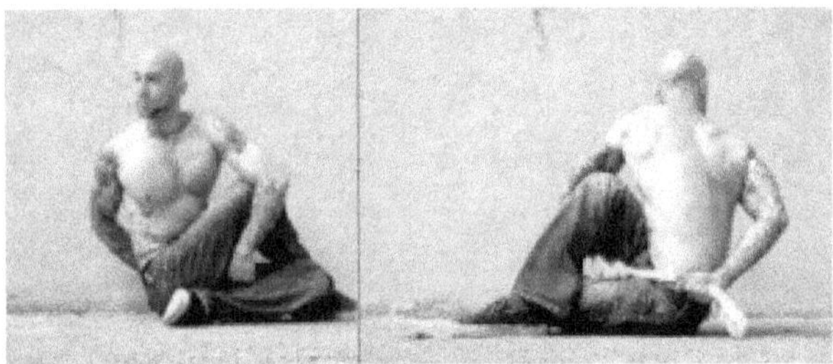

Each time you stretch, you will assume this position holding the towel in two hands. You will work your hands up and down the towel, slowly bringing your hands together by gripping greater portions of the towel. Eventually, you will be able to clasp fingers, and that is the final level of the twist stretch.

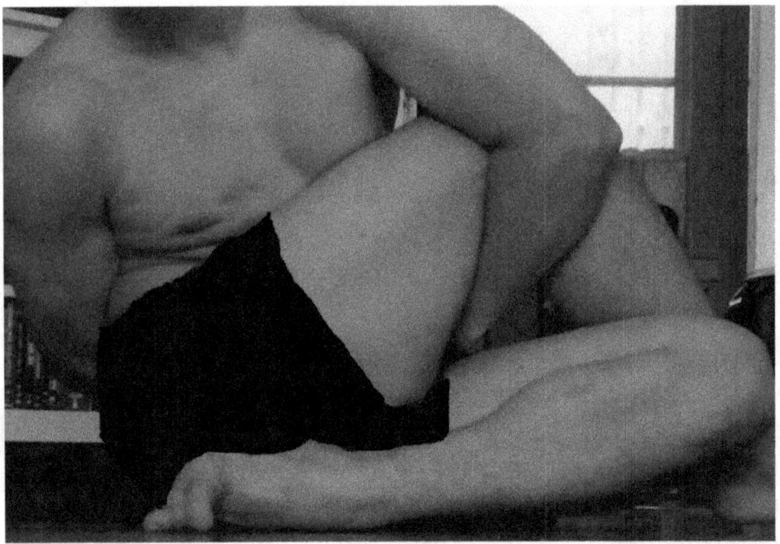

This process will be slow and arduous—it took me the better part of a year of consistent training to get my fingers to touch, but I have already noticed increased mobility, flexibility, and decreased back pain.

The towel stretch can be made easier by remembering to "worm" both hands up the towel, not just one. Actively use both to secure deeper stretches, and you will notice progress.

Doing even the easiest variations of this stretch will make you notice an immediate healing of the spine: your back will deliciously crack and you'll feel warm and limber afterwards. And with practicing the more advanced variants, you will make yourself more limber for whatever physical activity you engage in, ranging from dancing to getting out of submission holds.

But there's a lot more stretches you can work on, and these will be a few that you might recognize, such as...

1. The Bow Stance

This works the hip flexors, making your hips more mobile and flexible. Put one leg behind the other, as far as it can go while keeping the back foot flat on the floor. Keep the chest and back straight and vertical. Bend the front leg, go until parallel. Keep pressure on the back leg. The stretch is felt in the hip and groin, and as always the back is kept high and straight. Switch legs when done.

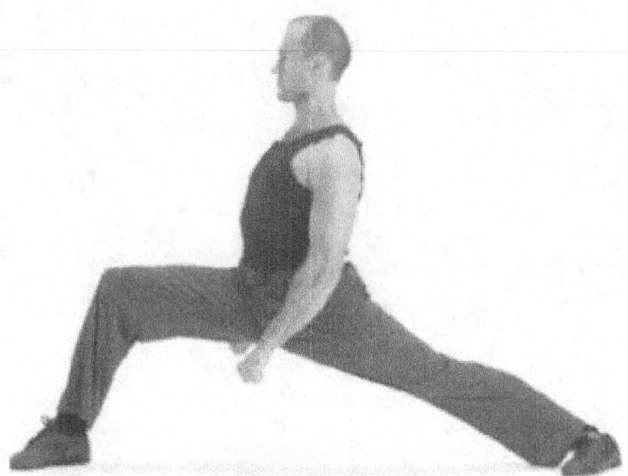

2. The Floor Hamstring Stretch

This is one we all remember from elementary school. Sit down on the floor, and extend your legs fully. Keep the feet together and pointed straight up, keep the chest and back high and straight, and bend at the waist, reaching your arms to your feet. I say "arms" and not "hands," because training can enable you to reach your hands beyond your feet, as seen in the picture.

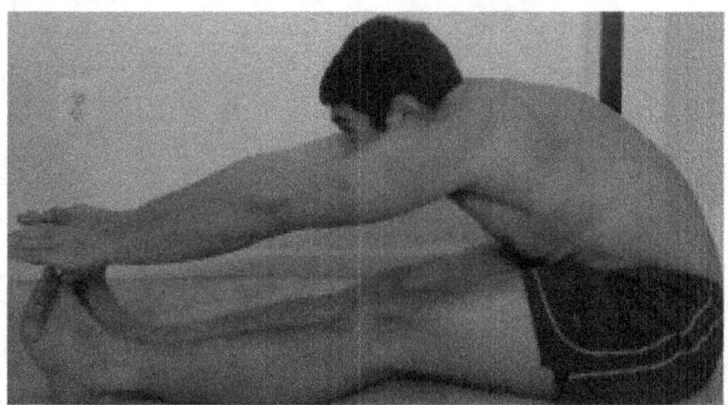

3. The Hang Stretch

One of two stretches I do after weightlifting (the other being the bridge), which I will admit is somewhat hypocritical of me, but you'll realize why when you do the stretch. Hang from a pull-up bar, with arms fully extended and the breath held, then, let the breath go in one gasp, and let your body sag. You should feel the stretch in the back muscles. Helps your posture as well.

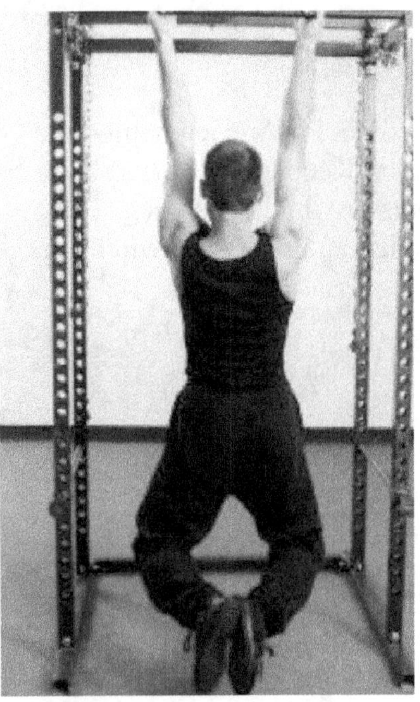

4. The Chest Stretch

Put your feet together and stand straight. Then clench the buttocks and thrust the hips forward, while keeping your back as straight as possible, lean your head back and look at the ceiling, and spread your arms out and as wide as possible (do NOT lock the elbows). This expands the chest and shoulders, reduces "droopiness" of the neck, and reduces hyperlordosis in the lumbar as well.

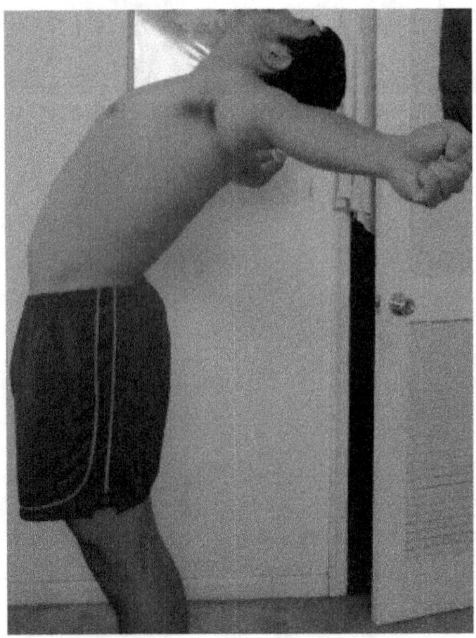

5. The Floor Hip Flexor Stretch

Put one foot on the ground, and one knee on the ground far behind. Then lean forward on the front leg, keeping the back and chest high and straight (I repeat, do not move your torso at all), while putting pressure on the hind leg. You should feel the stretch in the hip flexor of the hind leg. Then switch legs and repeat

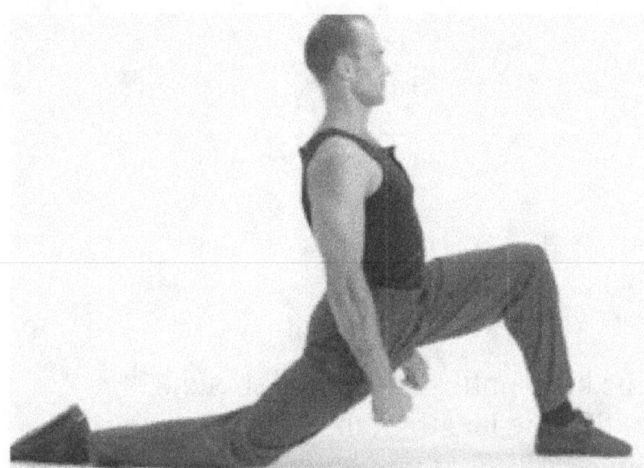

These stretches, combined with bridging, will deal with the overwhelming majority of your joint and muscle pains. But if you really want to get a good workout with stretching, and I mean *really* get the sweat pouring and your heart pounding, then you're going to have to work on that nigh-impossible feat known as the splits.

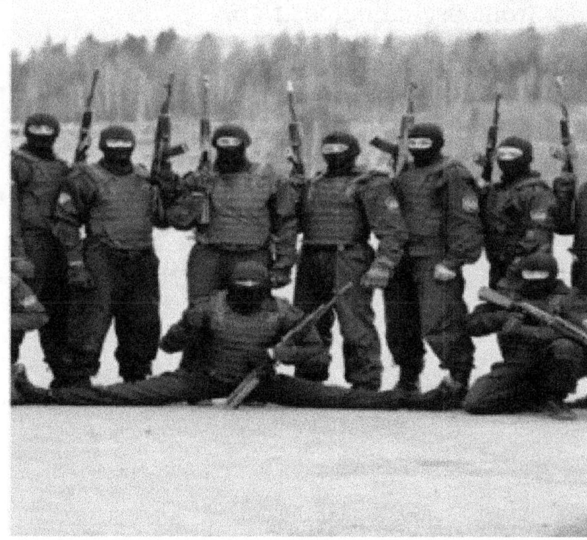

Spetsnaz can't be wrong!

Obviously, you are not going to go from stiff legs to split immediately---and this is where you're going to have to relax into the stretch, as you have learned.

There are two split to train---the front split and the side split. The front split is easier so we'll be doing that first.

To begin, wear long sweatpants and socks. Get into the kneeling hip flexor position, and then slide the front foot forward until it is totally straight.

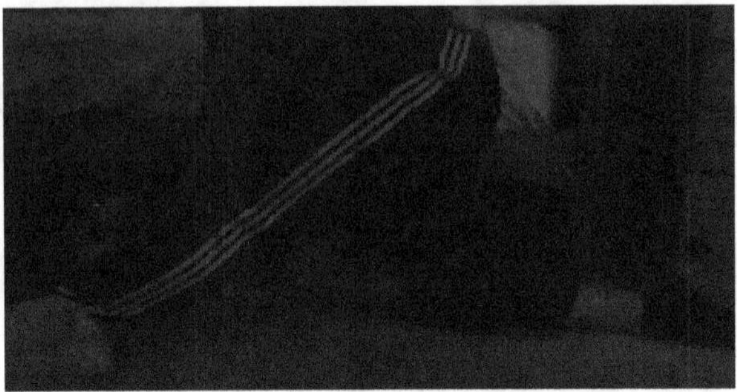

Then slide the legs apart with the hind leg sliding on its knee until you feel the stretch. Remember your PNF and relaxation techniques. I feel that the length of the hold is more important than forcing the stretch. In other words, doing 75-80% of your maximum stretch and holding that for 20 minutes is better than doing 100% of your maximum and only holding it for 1 minute.

Over the course of many training sessions, try to spread your legs apart farther and farther until you are doing the front split.

The side split is done similarly, sliding your feet apart from a standing position.

With all the information given in the exercise chapter, you will be well on your way to losing weight. But you're not there yet---because you have not yet utilized the "secret weapon" for weight loss. And that will come...right now!

Chapter 5: Informal Exercise: The Weight Loss Secret

You've heard me mention this mysterious term "informal exercise" more than once in this book. So now you must be asking what the hell *is* "informal exercise"?

To explain what it is, I have to explain what it <u>isn't</u>: informal exercise is not, as you might imagine, a period where you put on specially designated exercise clothes and set a goal of time/intensity to exercise. Nor is it a period where you'll be in pain and under great toil (huzzah!)

No, informal exercise is by definition done very mildly and relaxed, and more often than not in street clothes. It encompasses things such as walking, leisurely bicycling, dancing, and other non-intensive activities. However, the key is that informal exercise has to be done *in conjunction with formal exercise* for maximum results!

How can you mix both of these into your busy schedule? It's quite simple---do informal exercise not for its own sake, but for the sake of accomplishing some of those goals in your busy life. For example, do you have a letter to drop off at the post office? Don't drive---walk there! Have another appointment? Bike there! And so forth. As a rule of thumb, if the round trip is less than 5 miles---walk. If it's between 5 and 10 miles---bike.

Without even knowing it (and without any strenuous effort), a 2 mile walk will burn you an extra 200 calories---and since that's 10% of your daily caloric needs, combining that with a regimented and structured exercise program will show you big results pretty quick. Plus, you got your errands done.

Alternatively, do an active, yet leisurely activity like dancing on the same day as your workout. That'll burn an extra hundred calories or two.

Indeed, this concept of informal exercise is probably the most peasant-y aspect of this peasant's diet: I discovered this secret back in college, purely to save money on bus/subway fare when I was going out and about town (*ahem* and by "going out on the town" I of course mean "sleeping with every woman I could find..."), but quickly found that I was losing weight without even realizing it. Similarly, your hearty yeoman ancestors hoofed it everywhere and anywhere, because it's not like they could afford a horse or any other form of transportation.

Remember: Eat to save money and transport yourself to save money, and weight loss will become yours without you ever realizing it---until you suddenly wake up and realize you've dropped a few jeans sizes.

The reason I specify that the informal exercise has to be light and leisurely is due to the simple fact that if you engage in a more strenuous form of exercise, you might tire yourself out for your formal exercise---and a half-assed workout benefits nobody.

As a side note, "informal exercise" will, I find, reduce your soreness from the formal workout. To cite one example, back in my aforementioned college days, I would lift weights and then afterwards walk a couple of miles to the off-campus apartment of a young lady that I would, er, play Parcheesi with. The leisurely walk to and from her quarters, combined with the sweaty voluptuousness of a vigorous game of Parcheesi, would leave me feeling remarkably fresh and un-sore the next morning.

In short, that's how to maximize your exercise results: just move more! Use your own better judgment of course to avoid muscle tear or injury, and within a month or two you'll see results. You *were* planning on getting a month older, weren't you?

The information I have provided you up to this point should help you with your weight loss and fitness goals...but wait! You still have some questions! So let's answer them!

Let me just say that as a personal trainer I am so goddamn tired of hearing this. Like, a lot. So I'm going to put this to pat right now for any women that are reading this book:

YOU ARE A WOMAN. YOU DO NOT HAVE THE BIOCHEMICAL EQUIPMENT TO GET BIG MANLY MUSCLES.

Excuse me for shouting. I'll be gentler now---but yes, the basic argument was encapsulated in that loud cloddish statement. You are a woman, and unless you've made the *terrible* mistake of getting a PhD in cultural anthropology you have likely noticed throughout your life that you are somewhat different from a man.

Men, by nature of being men, produce hormones called androgens from the time they start gestating in the womb---androgens being a wonderful little chemical cocktail of virility, muscularity, and poor decision making.

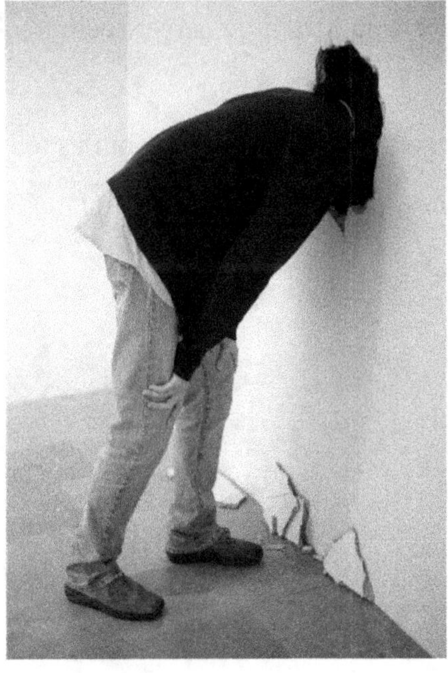

Testosterone!

In all seriousness, the presence of these hormones, most predominantly testosterone, leads to the secondary sexual characteristics that we associate with masculinity in both its most glorious and most buffoonish forms:

- Increased bone density and size
- Increased muscle mass
- Deeper voices
- Increased hirsuteness
- Increased spatial reasoning and overall "right-braindedness"

But also...

- Increased violent tendencies
- Increased sex drive
- And most damningly "conspicuous bravery" (ie: foolhardiness and bravado that on rare occasions leads to scientific/technological breakthroughs and/or world record breaking stunts but mainly leads to young men getting themselves killed doing stupid things).

The female body does produce testosterone but in much smaller numbers, which is why women are indeed smaller and more physically weak on average than a man, but also less likely to commit crime or get themselves killed doing some stupid "hold my beer" stunt. Or as Camille Paglia once wrote, "there are no female Mozarts for the same reason there's no female Jack the Ripper". So to put it in another words, you won't get big manly muscles unless you're giving yourself manly hormones---just stay away from steroids and you'll be fine!

With all that being said, I can't help but feel that the sorts of long and lithe and elegant muscles that women tend to want would be better accomplished by calisthenics rather than weight training. At the very least, the women that I have trained in my personal training career seem to respond to, and enjoy, calisthenics more so than weights.

Try for yourself and see what works for you---both exercise "genres" will be effective, but as to your personal preference, only you can decide!

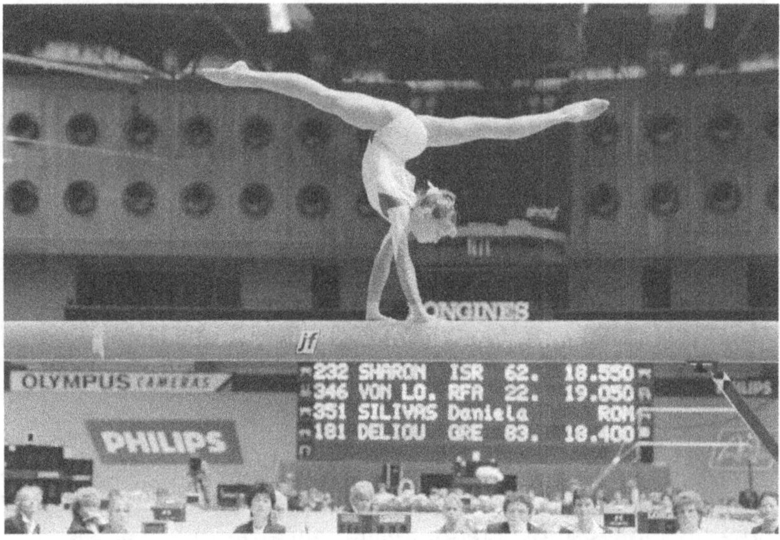

No weights were used to make this body

Chapter 7: What programming should I use?

You already should have a basic grasp on "programming" by reading my discussion of what days you should do what type of exercise, but this chapter will go into greater detail about types of programming to achieve certain goals. As a rule of thumb, most discussions of programming will revolve around resistance training, as the other forms of exercise are very simple in comparison.

And now for a few examples of programming for specific goals:

Should you simply want to achieve the very femme fitness goal of "toning up" your muscles without adding bulk, you are going to want to lift heavy weights with EXTREMELY low repetitions. By "extremely low repetitions", I mean like 2 or 3 repetitions <u>at most</u>. All of the resistance exercises I discussed with you must be done with those low repetitions: every lift and every step of the calisthenic progressions. When you can do 2-3 reps with the weight you're working with, or the calisthenic step you're working on, then move on. This is also sufficient purely to lose weight.

If, however, you want to bulk up and add muscle mass...then you're probably a man. In that case, sir, you will want to lift slightly less heavy weights and higher repetitions. And I emphasize "slightly" less heavier---whereas the extremely low repetitions in the preceding paragraph should be done with a weight that taxes 100% of your strength capacity, this should be in the 85-90% range. In other words, if your maximum squat is 300 pounds, you would do 1-2 reps of 300 if you just wanted to build "lean strength", but you would do 5-10 reps of 275-280 (broken up into sets) if you wanted to build size.

There are two types of hypertrophy (muscle size): myofibrillar (where you have an increased number of muscles fibers) and sarcoplasmic (where the amount of cytosol within the cell membrane of an individual muscle fiber increases)

Initial Muscle   Myofibrillar Hypertrophy   Sarcoplasmic Hypertrophy

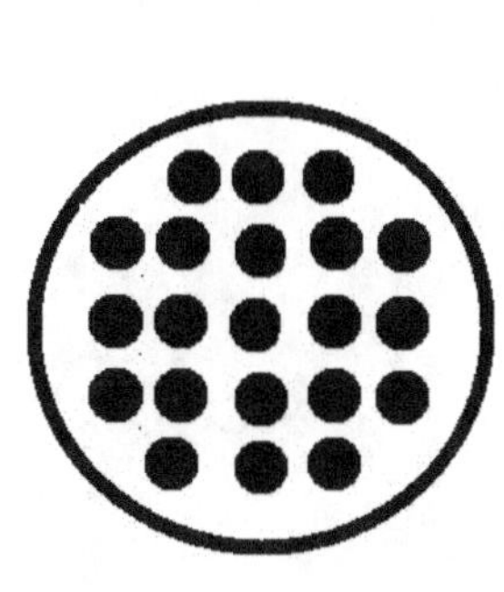

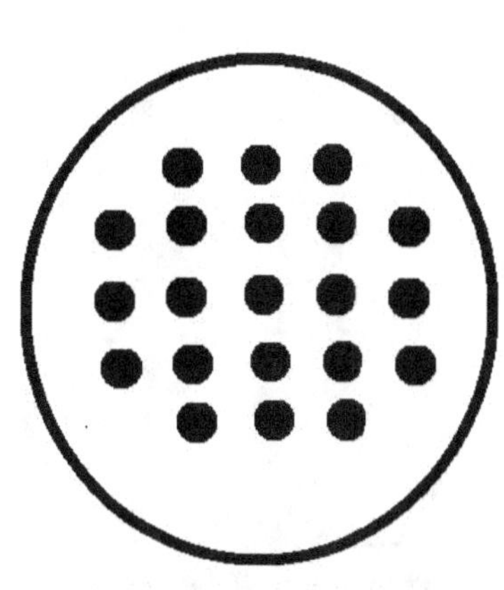

Functional hypertrophy - the contractile elements of the muscle cell are bigger

Non-Functional Hypertrophy - The cell is bigger but the contractile elements remain at the same size

Very simplified, of course

The former is the only one that will actually make you stronger, but of course being able to look muscular *without* having to take your clothes off is its own reward---the more of your maximal capacity you utilize the more myofibrillar hypertrophy you will develop, but of course you cannot do many repetitions of your maximal capacity---by virtue of it *being* your maximal lift, you will exhaust yourself very quickly.

Thus, sarcoplasmic hypertrophy involves doing lesser weight and more repetitions. And the smarter reader is probably thinking to themselves "Wait a minute...if I can get bigger muscles by doing 5-10 reps of 85-90% capacity...then what if I do 20-30 reps of 50% capacity, or 50 reps of 25%, or 100 reps with an unloaded bar?!"

Those will indeed give you sarcoplasmic hypertrophy...and they'll also give you useless Potemkin Village muscles (to borrow Pavel Tsatsouline's phraseology). And no humble yeoman would be able to plow his acreage or pull his longbow if he has big useless fluffy muscles---I'd stick with no more than 10 reps to get both hypertrophy and functional ability.

Chapter 8: Roam On, Yeoman

Do you see how simple that was? Less than 100 pages, and you have all the information you need to lose weight and have all the nutrients you need to build muscles. Putting food in your mouth and exercising are quite literally the simplest things you can possible do---and yes, I *am* implying that if you can't do it, you're failing your hardscrabble ancestors.

Yeomen and serfs and peasants, habitual farmers and occasional conscripted infantrymen thrust into a maelstrom of cold iron with naught but a "padded jack" shirt and a spear, desperate to survive and thrive (because who doesn't want to get the day off from work on Walpurgis Night?) And the fact that you're standing here right now quite obviously shows that they survived long enough to have kids. And those kids had to survive scarlet fever and measles and mumps and tuberculosis long enough to have kids themselves, and so forth until you were born.

You have many, *many* advantages over your ancestors, and yet you still aren't a tenth of the person they are (well, in the literal sense you're probably at least twice the person they are---- wakka wakka!)

In seriousness, it's time to fix that problem, don't you think? *Ville Gagnee! Deus le Vult!* And eat on!

APPENDIX: A Basic Meal Plan

As a personal trainer, I have worked in various gyms that do consultations and meal plan consulting for the training clients. I have taken one of those meal plans and modified it enough to not get sued. Said meal plan consists of what foods to buy; combine this with the "palm of your hand" eating regimen above, and marvel at your weight loss!

...Of course, if you TRULY are an impoverished peasant, just realize that it is possible to get every single vital nutrient if you eat sufficient quantities of milk and potatoes (with skins, not mashed or otherwise altered). But seeing as you'd probably go insane from monotony if you had to eat baked potatoes and milk for every meal every day, I wouldn't recommend this unless you are really that poor. For those of you that aren't so poor, here's a list of recommended foods

VEGETABLES

- ☐ ASPARAGUS
- ☐ BROCCOLI
- ☐ BRUSSELS SPROUTS
- ☐ CARROTS
- ☐ CUCUMBERS
- ☐ GARLIC
- ☐ GINGER
- ☐ LETTUCE
- ☐ KALE
- ☐ MUSHROOMS
- ☐ ONIONS
- ☐ PEPPERS
- ☐ SPINACH
- ☐ SWEET POTATOES
- ☐ TOMATOES
- ☐ ZUCCHINI
- ☐ STRING BEANS
- ☐ KIDNEY BEANS
- ☐ BLACK BEANS
- ☐ PUMPKIN
- ☐ SQUASH
- ☐ CHICKPEAS
- ☐ GREEN BEANS
- ☐ BEETS
- ☐ VEGIE BURGERS

NUTS & SEEDS

- ☐ ALMOND BUTTER
- ☐ ALMONDS
- ☐ CASHEWS
- ☐ PEANUT BUTTER
- ☐ PECANS
- ☐ PINE NUTS
- ☐ PUMPKIN SEEDS
- ☐ SESAME SEEDS
- ☐ WALNUT BUTTER
- ☐ WALNUTS
- ☐ MIXED NUTS
- ☐ PISTACHIOS
- ☐ HAZEL NUTS
- ☐ PEANUTS

FRUIT

- ☐ APPLES
- ☐ BANANAS
- ☐ BLUEBERRIES
- ☐ LEMONS
- ☐ LIMES
- ☐ MELON
- ☐ NECTARINES
- ☐ ORANGES
- ☐ PEACHES
- ☐ PEARS
- ☐ GRAPEFRUIT
- ☐ BLACK BERRIES
- ☐ RASPBERRIES
- ☐ STRAWBERRIES
- ☐ AVOCADO
- ☐ CHERRIES
- ☐ GRAPES
- ☐ CANTALOUPE
- ☐ RAISINS

OIL & VINEGAR

- ☐ APPLE CIDER VINEGAR
- ☐ BALSAMIC VINEGAR
- ☐ COCONUT BUTTER
- ☐ COCONUT OIL
- ☐ COOKING SPRAY
- ☐ EXTRA VIRGIN OLIVE OIL
- ☐ GRAPESEED OIL
- ☐ 5 RICE WINE VINEGAR
- ☐ ESAME OIL
- ☐ WHITE WINE VINEGAR

SWEETENERS

- ☐ AGAVE NECTAR
- ☐ HONEY
- ☐ JELLY
- ☐ PURE MAPLE SYRUP

SPICES

- ☐ BASIL
- ☐ BLACK PEPPER
- ☐ CAYENNE PEPPER
- ☐ CINNAMON
- ☐ CRUSHED RED PEPPER
- ☐ CUMIN
- ☐ GARLIC POWDER
- ☐ GROUND GINGER
- ☐ ITALIAN SEASONING
- ☐ NUTMEG
- ☐ ONION POWDER
- ☐ SEA SALT
- ☐ VANILLA EXTRACT

POULTRY & SEAFOOD & MEAT

- ☐ GRASS-FED BEEF
- ☐ GROUND TURKEY
- ☐ SALMON
- ☐ COD
- ☐ SEA BASS
- ☐ SNAPPER
- ☐ TUNA
- ☐ SCALLOPS
- ☐ SHRIMP
- ☐ CHICKEN BREAST
- ☐ GRILLED CHICKEN
- ☐ TURKEY
- ☐ DUCK

PANTRY STAPLES

- ☐ ANNIE'S SOUP
- ☐ BLACK BEANS
- ☐ COCONUT MILK
- ☐ GARBANZO BEANS
- ☐ KIDNEY BEANS
- ☐ VEGETABLE BROTH

GRAINS

- ☐ BROWN RICE
- ☐ BROWN RICE PASTA
- ☐ QUINOA
- ☐ QUICK-COOKING OATS
- ☐ OAT MEAL
- ☐ WHOLE WHEAT BREAD
- ☐ WHOLE WHEAT COUSCOUS
- ☐ WHOLE WHEAT PASTA
- ☐ WHOLE WHEAT TORTILLAS
- ☐ BULGUR (Cracked Wheat)

SWEETENERS

- ☐ AGAVE NECTAR
- ☐ HONEY
- ☐ JELLY
- ☐ PURE MAPLE SYRUP

SUPER FOODS

- ☐ CACAO NIBS
- ☐ CHIA SEEDS
- ☐ FLAX SEEDS

DAIRY

- ☐ EGGS/EGG WHITES
- ☐ FAT-FREE GREEK YOGURT
- ☐ UNSWEETENED ALMOND MILK

---

[i] Durant, Will, *The Age of Faith*

[ii] http://blogs.reuters.com/great-debate/2013/08/29/why-a-medieval-peasant-got-more-vacation-time-than-you/

[iii] McCallister, Peter, *Manthropology*